THE COUNTRYSIDE COOKBOOK

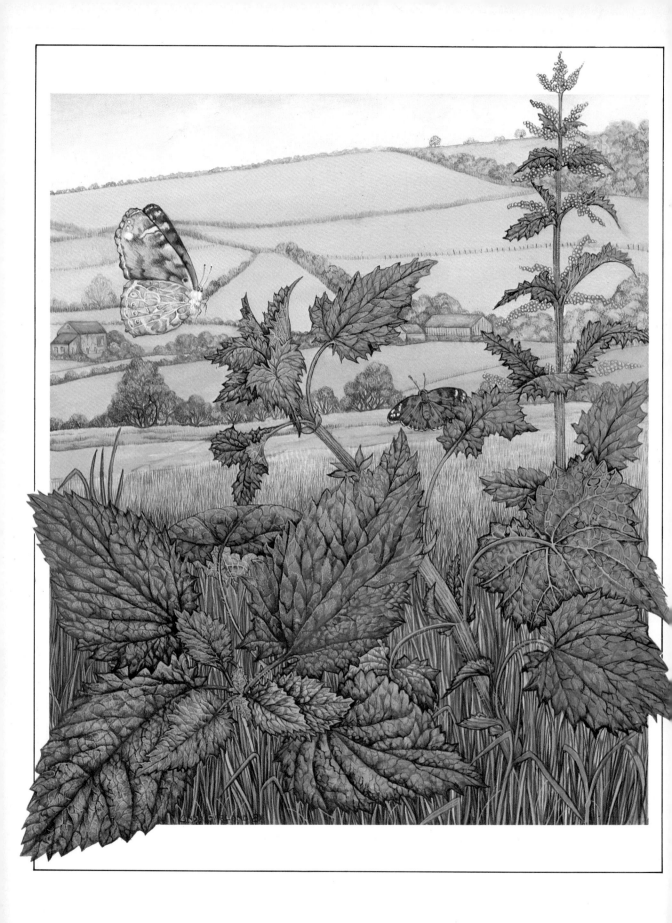

THE COUNTRY-SIDE COOK BOOK

Recipes & Remedies

GAIL DUFF

Illustrated by
LINDA GARLAND

with line illustrations by

ROGER GARLAND

VNR VAN NOSTRAND REINHOLD COMPANY

NEW YORK   CINCINNATI   TORONTO   LONDON   MELBOURNE

THE COUNTRYSIDE COOKBOOK

Copyright © 1982 by Gail Duff, Linda and Roger Garland

Library of Congress Catalog Card Number 81-21920

ISBN 0-442-22084-7

Published in the United States in 1982
by Van Nostrand Reinhold Company
135 West 50th Street
New York, NY 10020, U.S.A.

Van Nostrand Reinhold Limited
1410 Birchmount Road
Scarborough, Ontario M1P 2E7, Canada

Published by agreement with Prism Press
Dorchester, Dorset, Great Britain

Designed by Mike Jarvis

Library of Congress Cataloging in Publication Data

Duff, Gail.
  The countryside cookbook.

  1. Cookery (Wild foods)   2. Wild plants, Edible.
I. Title.
TX823.D78   641.6   81–21920
ISBN 0–442–22084–7   AACR2

Printed and bound in Great Britain by Purnell and Sons,
Paulton, Bristol.

CONTENTS

For Maggie
Paula
and Stephen,
who put
up with
it all

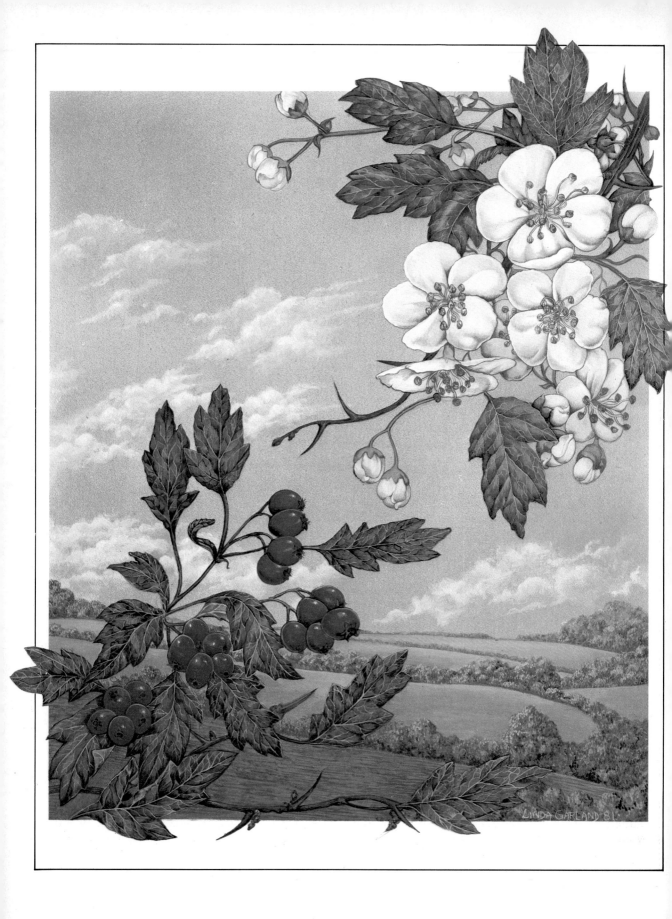

INTRODUCTION

The use of wild plants for food, drink and medicine, although enjoying a current vogue, is certainly nothing new. Indeed, if you look back far enough wild foods were once man's only foods, and even when farming and crop-growing had become accepted practise, berries, nuts and herbs were always used to supplement and flavour.

If you are a gardener, you will probably have found that there are certain periods in the spring when you come to the end of one crop and are waiting for another to start. Now we can go out to the supermarket to buy something imported to fill in the gap, but this is only a recent innovation. In a time when both farmer and cottager relied only on home grown produce which probably ran out quickly during the harsh winter weather, what more natural than to go out into field and hedgerow to pick Nature's early leaves? As well as satisfying hunger and adding flavour to the pottage pot, the vitamins and minerals that they contain helped, in Culpeper's words, to 'cleanse the blood in spring' and to keep away scurvy. Later in the year, there would be more leaves and other delicacies which only Nature can provide such as wild strawberries, the different kinds of seaweeds and wild mushrooms. Cultivated mushrooms are a twentieth-century convenience, but even so, no one has ever successfully cultivated a Cep or a Chanterelle. Even the Paris markets and London's Dorchester Hotel have to rely on wild ones from European forests.

What would we do without coffee and tea? They have become universal beverages to be found in almost every western home. But until the seventeenth century we had never even heard of them and although they then became rapidly popular with the upper classes in towns and cities, they reached the countryside only rarely, and even in the big houses were treated as something for special occasions rather than drinks to be consumed several times a day. Country people drank what we now call herb teas or tisanes, made from leaves and herbs which grew in cottage gardens and which could be gathered along the hedgerows. They were made in the same way as ordinary tea and served without milk, sweetened occasionally with honey. Even when tea became more readily available at the end of the nineteenth century, only a little could be afforded in the homes of the agricultural workers and it was still very much supplemented with dried wild leaves such as chamomile, mint and blackberry leaves.

Herb and leaf teas have a wide variety of soft, gentle flavours which can be so much more pleasant than the harsh teas that so often fill tea bags. They are also more healthy to drink regularly than tea or coffee since they do not contain caffeine. You can buy herb teas in packets and sachets but how much more satisfying to make your own.

Herbal teas were not the only drink. There was nearly always a jar of beer in the house. It was not strong, but more like a weak mild ale and it was brewed in the home kitchen. Hops, which are now universally used to flavour and preserve beer, generally came into use in the sixteenth century. Before this, we all drank ale made only from malted barley, yeast and water flavoured with bitter herbs. It was mostly the brewers who used hops when they were first introduced. The poor could rarely afford to buy them and for many years they continued to use the old herbal knowledge, using whatever flavouring leaves that were in season such as dandelions or broom tops in the spring and burdock in late summer. Herb beers are light, not very strong and very refreshing, just right for quenching your thirst during a hard day's work in field or garden.

The country woman also made wine, and her ingredients were garden fruits and flowers and berries that she gathered from the countryside. They were fermented in large earthenware crocks with yeast and sugar. Home brewing is now undergoing a new-found popularity and although you can buy canned concentrates, the fruits, berries and flowers are still there for the picking.

Doctor's prescriptions and pharmacists to make them up have not always been conveniently to hand and so until the beginning of the present century every country housewife had to know which herbs and plants would cure the everyday illnesses of her family and also of the animals. She knew where to find the plants, which parts to use and how to prepare them. It came as natural to her as reaching for the bottle of aspirins or demanding a doctor's prescription does to us today, and in many cases the cure was just as effective. There were no side effects and no resistance was built up to the remedies to make them ineffectual in times of real need. Herbal remedies are simple to make and to take, and a cupboard full of dried herbs makes a safe medicine chest.

Gathering from the fields for cooking, flavouring, brewing and curing was a natural way of life for all country people for centuries. They even gave the plants local names such as Sauce Alone, Scarwort or Baccy Plant which indicates how they were commonly known and used. When we came to the twentieth century, however, life changed. Somehow, with two world wars to cope with, the gradual increase of the convenience food market and the ease with which patent medicines could be obtained, everyone forgot that the countryside yields a wealth of useable plants throughout the year. Two generations later, the tide is turning again. Natural medicines and foods are being rediscovered and in many cases are being found after all to be better for us than the chemical and the refined.

So here is the Countryside Cookbook, full of simple remedies and easy recipes, made with plants that everyone can gather.

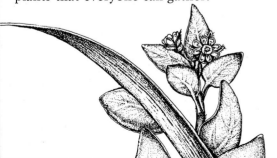

Harvesting

Equipment

When you are going out on a picking expedition, there are various things that will make life easier. The most important piece of equipment is probably a good pair of rubber boots. They will keep your feet warm and dry and also prevent your legs and feet from being scratched by thorns or stung by nettles.

If you are picking nettles, then take a pair of rubber gloves. Gardening gloves are useful if you are going to pick anything with thorns.

A walking stick or shepherd's crook is handy when you have to reach up into trees or across bushes. With it, you can pull the branches towards you without breaking them.

An open basket is probably the best container for wild foods, especially nuts, berries, mushrooms and large quantities of leaves. For very juicy berries such as blackberries or ripe elderberries, line the basket with plastic to stop the juice from dripping through. When you are picking leaves on a very windy day, have something in the basket to anchor them down. It can be very frustrating to see all your crop disappear over the next hedge! Most plastic bags can be used for leaves, and also for the nuts and drier berries as long as you don't leave them in the bag for too long. But never use plastic for mushrooms. They will sweat and you will end up with a soggy and unappetising mess.

When you only pick a bunch of flowers or herbs, wrap the ends of the stems in damp paper towels and then in a plastic bag to keep them fresh on the way home.

If you want a volume measure of flowers for wine, it helps if you pick them directly into a measured container, such as a plastic bucket. Put small amounts of single flower heads like broom into a plastic bag and remember that some flowers like daisies will close after having been picked for about 30 minutes and if you want to use them as a garnish you should rush to the kitchen with them immediately.

Seaweeds can be put into plastic bags, but they do tend to leak, so a plastic bucket is probably better.

You will need a pair of good quality scissors when gathering things like watercress, herbs and nettles; and you must have a good sharp knife for cutting the ends off mushroom stalks.

Location

There is no doubt about it, the countryside these days is shrinking. Farming is also becoming more intensive, and, regrettably, there are very few meadows full of summer flowers just waiting to be picked. So you might have to look a little harder for plants than you might have done only twenty years ago.

Patches of deciduous woodland contain many edible species, and the grassy clearings within them and the areas immediately around them are also good hunting places. You can find a great many plants along the verges and banks beside country lanes, but it is best not to choose busy roads where the traffic and fumes are likely to be high. Heath and patches of public land contain their own particular species and waste ground is quite prolific, although some of the plants there could be on the scrubby side if the soil is poor.

If you see just what you want growing in someone's garden, knock on the door and ask for his permission before you go in, even if it is only for a few dandelion leaves. You never know, the owners may be wanting to eat them too!

The same applies to farmland. Never go marauding across fields or through orchards without asking the farmer's permission. Farmland is not common property, it is one man's means of obtaining a livelihood. Once you have permission, be careful of growing crops and remember that it is wild foods that you are out for and not a stolen apple.

Be careful, when you are on farmland, that you do not pick from an area that has recently been sprayed or your plants will be contaminated.

If you take your dog with you, make sure he stays with you. Tether him to a fence, if necessary, and make him wait. Never take a dog into a field containing sheep and young lambs, and if you walk through a field of grown sheep, keep him on a lead.

Time

The best picking weather is dry weather. You will be more comfortable and your harvest in better condition. When picking leaves, nuts or berries you can really choose your time of day. Flowers and herbs should be picked on a dry morning, after the dew has gone but before the sun is really hot.

Identification

Always take field guides out with you and never pick anything about which you are doubtful. This applies especially to mushrooms.

Picking

If you are in a good area for a particular plant, the chances are that you will find not only one patch of it but many. Do not, therefore, pick the whole of one clump of flowers, just pick a few from each. When picking berries or nuts, go from tree to tree always leaving a few. You can, however, safely pick every mushroom that you see since the main body of the plant is spread underground in a large network.

If you find only one example of any of the other species, then leave it alone and perhaps by the following year it will have increased to a clump.

Only pick the best specimens of any species. That way you will taste them at their best and obtain the optimum medicinal values.

Always ensure that you leave the countryside still looking attractive, still able to feed wild animals such as squirrels and able to supply more food for you to gather next year.

Cleaning

On getting home, the first thing that most of your plants will need is a good rinse in cold water to clean and refresh them. Put them into a bowl of cold water, dunk them around for a bit and lift them out. If they are very gritty, rinse the bowl and repeat the process. Never leave your plants submerged in cold water as this destroys vitamins.

Drying Plants and Herbs

Make sure that the plants and leaves are not damp when you pick them and dry them carefully since both flavour and medicinal properties can be lost in the process. The best time to pick for drying is just before the flowers appear.

The best place for drying small amounts of herbs is in an airing cupboard. Either tie them in bunches or lay them out in wire racks which you have previously covered with muslin. You can also put drying racks in an oven set at the lowest possible temperature. In warm weather you can use a warm, darkened room or an airy garden shed. Over the central heating boiler is another good place, provided it is not in a steamy room or in direct sunlight.

To dry seed heads, such as those of fennel, put them upside down into paper bags and tie the bags round the stems. Again hang them in the airing cupboard or a warm dry room until, when the bags are shaken, the seeds fall into the bottom.

When herbs are dry they should be crisp but still fairly bright green. Crumble them and pack them into air and light tight tins or jars. Do not keep dried herbs for longer than a year. After this their flavour and medicinal properties diminish rapidly.

Garden Cultivation

If you take a particular liking to any one of the wild plants you may want to establish it for convenience in your garden. Some, in fact, may already be there and just need a little cosseting. Provided you find a large patch of plants you can safely dig up one or two along with as much of their root system as possible and a clump of their surrounding earth.

If they are one of the rapidly spreading varieties such as ground elder or mint, grow them in a sunken bath or build a sunken wall of concrete blocks around them.

Wild roses can be grown by a wall or fence, hops up a frame and blackberries can be trained on wires in a fruit garden in a similar fashion to raspberries. Many wild nut and fruit trees can be bought from specialist garden centres and experimental growers.

I have tried in vain to scatter mushroom spores about, but they seem to have a mind of their own. If you have your own clear stream you can successfully transplant watercress and if you have a private beach you might even be able to experiment with seaweed!

The Plants

The plants we have chosen for this book are by no means the only edible species. They have been chosen for the following reasons:

1. They all grow in Britain, Scandinavia, Europe the United States, and many in Australasia.
2. None of them at the time of writing is scarce and picking them will not damage their ability to survive.
3. Of the more common plants, they are the most edible and useful.

The Recipes

I have tried to keep the recipes as simple as possible so that they can be used by every interested family besides the experienced cook. Many take only a short time to prepare since no one wants to spend hours in the kitchen after spending the day out picking.

Most of the recipes use only small amounts of a particular plant. This makes it easier in that you can pick what you need in a relatively short time. It is also better from a conservation point of view.

To save repetition in some of the recipes, here are some explanations of equipment and basic methods:

Jam and Jelly Making

Use fruit as fresh as possible, just on the point of ripeness and never over-ripe.

Bring the fruits to the boil in the required amount of water and simmer them gently until they are reduced to a pulp (about 45 minutes for jam and 1½ hours for jelly).

When making a jelly, strain the pulp through a scalded jelly bag and allow it to drain naturally without squeezing the bag. Leave it until the juice stops dripping through (this may take up to three hours) and finish the process as soon as possible after this. The strained liquid should be brought back to the boil before you add the sugar.

Granulated sugar is suitable for all jams and jellies, although lump or preserving sugars will give a brighter, clearer appearance.

Dark brown sugar may also be used successfully. It will not flavour the jam or jelly but will give it a very dark colour. The jam will set just as easily as with the white sugars.

Warming the sugar in a low oven before adding it to the jam or jelly will make it dissolve quicker.

When the sugar is added, stir until it has dissolved and let the jam or jelly boil without stirring.

To test for setting point:

1. Check with a thermometer, having warmed it in water first. A temperature of 105–110C (220–222F) is required for adequate setting.

2. Drop 5 ml (1 teaspoon) jam or jelly on to a cool plate. The surface should set and crinkle if you push it with your finger.

3. See how the jam drips from a wooden spoon—it should break off cleanly in flakes.

When setting point is reached, take the jam or jelly from the heat and skim it.

Pour it into sterilized glass jars or pots that have been warmed in the oven and fill them to the top.

After filling, lay a circle of waxed paper, waxed side down, on top. Cover the jars with a clean tea-cloth until the jam or jelly is completely cool.

When cool, seal either with circles of dampened cellophane or with screw tops.

Brewing

If you are going to be brewing beer or wine regularly then it is worthwhile collecting a few simple pieces of equipment and keeping them only for that purpose:

a large pan which holds at least 4.6 litres (1 gallon) of water, and for the larger batches, one that holds just over 9.2 litres (2 gallons);

a large container such as a plastic bucket that will withstand boiling water;

large and small funnels;

a syphon;

575 ml (1 pint) bottles and well fitting caps for beer;

wine bottles, corks and a corker;

4.6 litre (1 gallon) jars with fermenting locks for wine.

Ingredients

Yeast—for brewing beer, you can quite successfully use dried granulated baker's yeast; or you can get special brewing yeasts from chemists and home-brew shops. The strength varies between types and the amount needed is usually indicated on the packet. For wine, use a special wine yeast, also available from chemists and specialist shops.

Yeast nutrient—this is added to wines and can be bought in home-brew shops. The amounts needed are on the packet.

Pectolase—this makes the wine clear and helps to break down the fruits. It comes in both powder and tablet form and again the amounts should be indicated.

Beer

The beer brewing process is always basically the same. The water is boiled with the flavouring ingredients and then strained into a container holding the sugar and malt extract and possible other flavourings. It must then be cooled to around blood heat or until it feels lukewarm. The yeast is sprinkled on top, the container covered and left until the yeast starts to froth. Then put the container into a warm place, such as in the airing cupboard or beside a constantly burning cooker. Within a few hours the yeast will be working furiously and will have formed a thick crust on top of the beer which stays for about two days. After this the froth will die down and become a thin layer of bubbles. On about the third day the top will look flat. This means that fermentation has stopped. Syphon off the beer, leaving all the yeasty sediment in the bottom of the container. Put the beer into clean bottles and add 2.5 ml (½ teaspoon) sugar per 575 ml (1 pint) to get it working again and make it lively. Seal the bottles with well-fitting caps and stand them in the cool until the beer clears (this will be about a week). Pour the beer out carefully, leaving the sediment in the bottom of the bottles.

Wine

When the wine is in the fermenting jar, the yeast carries on working and gradually produces a layer of sediment in the bottom of the jar. When this is thick (in about three weeks) syphon off the clear liquid in the top into another jar. Make a sugar syrup by boiling 1.8 kg (4 lbs) sugar with 1.15 litres (2 pints) water for 15 minutes. Take it from the heat and add 7.5 g (¼ oz) tartaric acid. Cool the syrup and top up the wine with it until it again measures 4.6 litres (1 gallon). This process is called racking. Wait until another layer of sediment forms and rack again, adding more syrup. When the third layer forms, syphon off the clear wine but add no more syrup. Add 2 campden tablets per 4.6 litres (1 gallon) to stop the yeast working. This time, cork the jars. Leave the wine until it is completely clear and syphon it off into sterilised bottles. Cork it and keep it for at least 6 months before opening.

The Remedies

All the remedies in the book are simply made and with all of them there is no danger of over-dosage. They are only for minor ailments many of which are common in every household.

If you suspect that you are seriously ill, do not attempt to diagnose and dose yourself without consulting a doctor. If you would rather not receive a conventional form of treatment then go to a qualified homeopathic doctor. Not everyone wishes to use herbal remedies, indeed, they may not work for everybody. It is nevertheless interesting to know about the traditional medicinal uses of everyday plants.

There are various ways of making herbal remedies which are repeated throughout the book. To save them from being too wordy, here are the basic methods:

Infusion. An infusion is made like a cup of tea. If a recipe says, for example, infuse the herb in 575 ml (1 pint) boiling water for 10 minutes you put the herb into a pot or jug, pour the boiling water on it, cover it and leave it for 10 minutes. Strain it before drinking. Each recipe will give the required amount of herb and water and the length of time to leave them.

Decoction. This is stronger than an infusion. The herb is put into a saucepan with cold water, brought to the boil and simmered either for a specified time or until the liquid has reduced to a specified amount. The liquid may be strained immediately or you may have to wait until it has cooled before straining. The exact method will be indicated.

Maceration. A maceration is produced by steeping a herb or plant in a cold liquid for a much longer time (12–24 hours).

Tincture. When a herb or plant is macerated in alcohol, the result is known as a tincture.

Useful information

1 American cup – 8 fl oz – 225 ml
1¼ American cups – 10 fl oz – ½ Imperial pint – 275 ml
2 American cups – 1 American pint – 16 fl oz – 425 ml
2½ American cups – 20 fl oz – 1 Imperial pint – 575 ml

Sugar: 1 American cup – 8 oz – 225 g
Flour: 1 American cup – 4 oz – 125 g

Throughout the book it is assumed that fresh herbs are available. If they are not available, use half the given amount of dried herbs.

SPRING

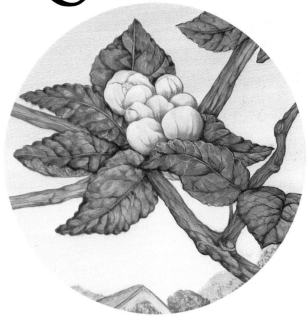

BROOM

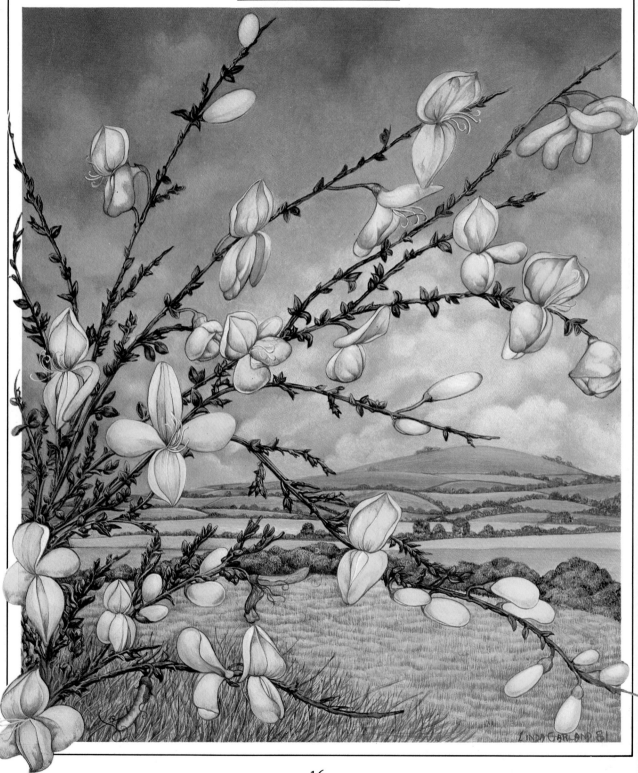

Linda Garland 81

Availability

Broom grows throughout Britain, Scandinavia and Europe. It is spreading increasingly in the United States, particularly in the eastern coastal regions. In Australia it is mainly found in gardens — not wild. Broom grows best on dry downs, sandy pastures and heaths and wasteland. The young green tops may be picked in early spring and again in the autumn and the buds and flowers through-out spring and early summer.

When using the flowers, use only the yellow parts as the green calyx tends to give a bitter flavour. Medicinally, both the leaves and flowers can be used fresh or dried.

Broom Sauce

This sauce is delicious poured over hard boiled eggs, white fish, grilled bacon, ham, or roast chicken or turkey.

25 g (1 oz) butter
30 ml (2 tablespoons) wholewheat flour
200 ml (7 fl oz) stock
90 ml (3 fl oz) dry white wine
90 ml (3 fl oz) broom flowers
30 ml (2 tablespoons) chopped parsley
sea salt and freshly ground black pepper

Melt the butter in a frying pan on a moderate heat. Stir in the flour and cook it for ½ minute. Stir in the stock and bring it to the boil. Add the wine, broom flowers, parsley and seasonings.

Cover the pan and simmer the sauce for 15 minutes. Serve it hot.

Saffron Chicken with Broom

Broom and saffron give a delicate flavour to a sauce for a poached chicken.

one 1.35–1.57 kg (3–3½ lb) roasting chicken
150 ml (¼ pint) broom flowers
1 onion, peeled and stuck with 4 cloves
1 carrot, roughly chopped
1 celery stick, roughly chopped
5 ml (1 teaspoon) black peppercorns
bouquet of parsley
1 bayleaf
1.5 ml (¼ teaspoon) saffron
pinch sea salt
25 g (1 oz) butter
30 ml (2 tablespoons) wholewheat flour
60 ml (4 tablespoons) chopped parsley

Put the chicken into a large saucepan with 30 ml (2 tablespoons) broom flowers, the onion, carrot, celery, peppercorns, bouquet of parsley and bay-leaf. Pour in water to cover the legs of the chicken and add the saffron and salt. Bring the water to the boil, cover and simmer the chicken for 50 minutes.

Lift out the chicken. Strain and reserve the stock. Melt the butter in a saucepan on a moderate heat. Stir in the flour and cook it for ½ minute. Stir in 275 ml (½ pint) of the stock. Bring it to the boil and cook, stirring, until you have a thick sauce. Stir in the remaining broom and the chopped parsley. Keep the sauce warm.

Take all the chicken meat from the bones and cut it into 2.5 cm (1 inch) dice. Fold it into the sauce and heat it through without letting it cook any further. Serve with a savoury rice or with boiled new potatoes.

Save the stock for the following soup. Serves 4.

Broom and Chicken Soup

850 ml (1½ pints) stock reserved from poaching the
  above chicken
any odd scraps of left-over chicken meat scraped from
  the bones
90 ml (6 tablespoons) broom flowers
25 g (1 oz) butter
2 large onions, finely chopped
30 ml (2 tablespoons) wholewheat flour
sea salt and freshly ground black pepper
1 bayleaf
90 ml (6 tablespoons) chopped parsley
150 ml (¼ pint) natural yoghurt

Melt the butter in a saucepan on a low heat. Stir in the onions and cook them until they are soft. Stir in the flour and cook it for ½ minute. Stir in the stock and bring it to the boil. Season and put in the bayleaf, parsley and broom. Simmer, uncovered, for 15 minutes.

Take the pan from the heat and cool the soup a little. Stir in the yoghurt and the reserved chicken scraps. Reheat very gently if necessary, but do not boil again. Serves 4.

Broom and Almond Custards

Broom flowers can also give a delicate flavour to sweet dishes such as these rich custards.

25 g (1 oz) butter
30 ml (2 tablespoons) corn flour (corn starch)
275 ml (½ pint) milk
3 egg yolks
30 ml (2 tablespoons) honey
50 g (2 oz) almonds, blanched and ground
90 ml (6 tablespoons) broom flowers

Heat the oven to Reg 6/200C/400F. Melt the butter in a saucepan on a moderate heat. Stir in the cornflour and cook it for ½ minute. Stir in the milk and keep stirring until you have a smooth, thick sauce.

Take the pan from the heat. Beat in the egg yolks, one at a time, and stir in the honey, almonds and broom flowers.

Divide the mixture between 4 individual soufflé dishes and bake the custards for 20 minutes so they are set and the tops are golden brown. Serve them hot. Serves 4.

Broom Beer

This is a very light beer, good to quench your thirst after working in the garden.

50 g (2 oz) green broom tops
4.6 litres (1 gallon) water
450 g (1 lb) malt extract
225 g (8 oz) light brown (demerara) sugar
15 g (½ oz) dried yeast
2.5 ml (½ teaspoon) light brown (demerara) sugar per 575 ml (1 pint) bottle

Boil the broom tops in 1.725 litres (3 pints) water for 10 minutes. Dissolve the malt and sugar in 1.15 litres (2 pints) warm water. Strain the broom liquid into the solution, reserving the broom. Boil the broom in a further 1.725 litres (3 pints) water, also for 10 minutes. Strain the liquid onto the rest. Cover and leave the liquid until it cools to blood heat.

Sprinkle the yeast on top and leave the beer in a warm place to ferment for three days (or until fermentation stops).

Rack off the beer and bottle it, adding 2.5 ml (½ teaspoon) sugar per 575 ml (1 pint). Seal tightly and leave the beer undisturbed until it is clear (about 1 week).

Broom Wine

Broom wine is pale yellow and fragrant.

2.3 litres (4 pints) broom flowers
4.6 litres (1 gallon) boiling water
225 g (8 oz) sultanas, minced
1.35 kg (3 lbs) sugar
thinly pared rinds and juice 3 lemons
thinly pared rinds and juice 1 orange
175 ml (6 fl oz) cold black tea
yeast
yeast nutrient

Put the flowers into a container and pour on the boiling water. Leave them for 3 days, covered, stirring every day.

Strain the liquid onto the sultanas, sugar, fruit rinds and juices and tea. Add the yeast nutrient and sprinkle the yeast on top. Leave the wine in a warm place for 1 week.

Strain it into a jar and fit a fermentation lock. Rack as the wine clears and bottle when fermentation is complete.

Leave for 1 year before opening.

Medicinal

Broom Salve for Chapped Hands

50 g (2 oz) broom flowers
200 g (7 oz) petroleum jelly

Put the petroleum jelly into a small casserole and melt it on a low heat. Stir in the broom flowers. Bring the mixture just to boiling point, stir well and cover. Put the casserole into a warm oven (Reg under ¼/70C/200F) for 4 hours.

Strain the salve quickly through muslin into a small pot. Cover it completely when it is cold and set.

A cardiac tonic: Make a decoction with 25 g (1 oz) dried broom flowers and 1 litre (1¾ pints) water, boiling it for 1 minute. Strain. Take two cupfuls per day.

For yellow jaundice and other kidney complaints: Infuse 30 ml (2 tablespoons) broom tops in 425 ml (¾ pint) boiling water for 15 minutes. Strain. Take 15 ml (1 tablespoon) night and morning.

For dropsy of cardiac origin: Infuse 25 g (1 oz) dried broom tops in 575 ml (1 pint) boiling water for 15 minutes. Strain. Take a wineglassful four times a day.

Or, infuse 10 ml (2 teaspoons) fresh or dried blossoms in 225 ml (8 fl oz) boiling water for 15 minutes. Strain. Drink this amount twice a day.

For minor heart palpitations: Drink 225 ml (8 fl oz) of either of the above infusions before breakfast and again last thing at night.

For bladder and kidney infections: Put 25 g (1 oz) broom tops and 15 g (½ oz) dandelion root into a saucepan with 575 ml (1 pint) water. Boil until the liquid is reduced by half, adding 15 g (½ oz) crushed juniper berries just before the end.

For proteinuria: For 1 week in the month, drink one cupful of the flower infusion three times a day after meals.

Veterinary

To prevent sheep from contracting foot rot, make sure the young tops of broom are included in their winter fodder.

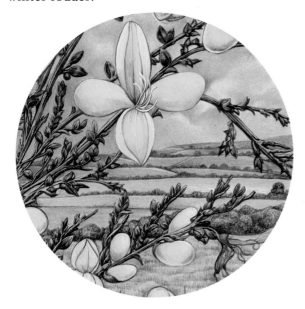

CHICKWEED

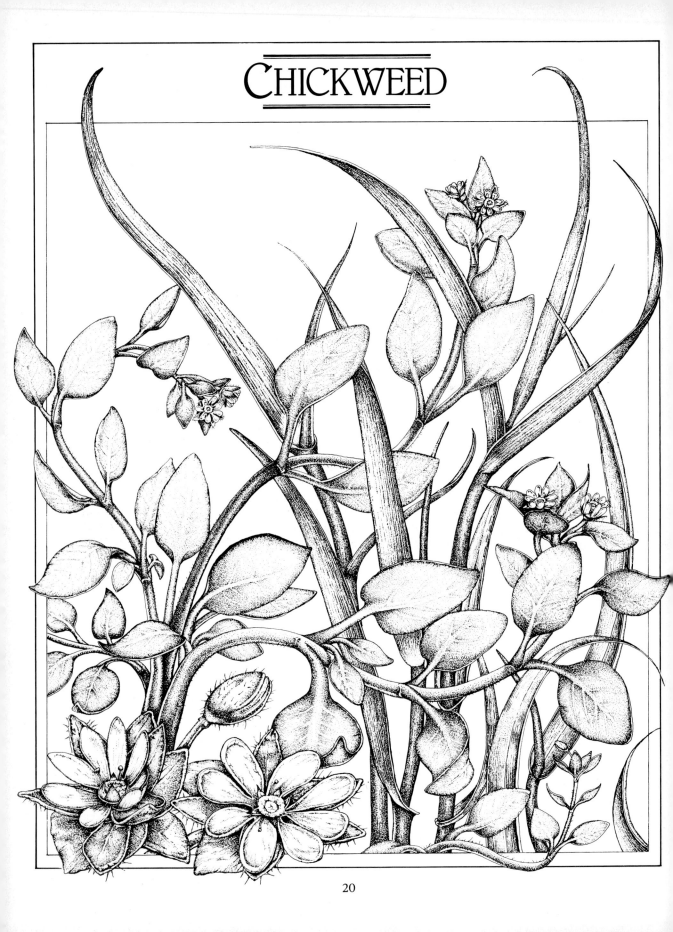

Availability

Chickweed grows all over the world, even in Northern Arctic regions. It flourishes best in open soil and the disturbed ground of gardens and fields.

If the weather is mild, chickweed might well be available for picking all through the winter, but it is at its most luxuriant in the spring and again in the autumn. When the small, starry white flowers first appear they can be cooked or eaten raw with the leaves and stems. Chickweed is not so palat-eable in the summer since the stems become longer and straggly. However, to use it medicinally, it is best picked in early summer (May to July in the northern hemisphere/September to February in Australasia).

Chickweed grows like a thick, green carpet so you can safely pull up handfuls of the stems and leaves without doing any harm. Before cooking or using medicinally, wash it well and trim off the stringy ends of the stalks as you would those of watercress. The weight given in the following recipes is that after the chickweed has been trimmed.

Chickweed Salad with Olives

Chickweed adds a fresh crispness to this spring salad. Serve it as a side dish with egg, cheese or fish dishes; or divide it between four small plates, scatter some chopped walnuts over the top and serve it as a first course.

50 g (2 oz) chickweed
50 g (2 oz) watercress
350 g (12 oz) tomatoes
2 medium oranges
12 black olives
60 ml (4 tablespoons) olive oil
30 ml (2 tablespoons) white wine vinegar
1 clove garlic, crushed with a pinch sea salt
freshly ground black pepper

Chop the chickweed and watercress. Chop the tomatoes. Peel and chop the oranges. Stone and quarter the olives. Mix all these in a salad bowl. Beat the remaining ingredients together and fold them into the salad.

Chickweed and Cheese Salad

Serve this salad as a first course.

40 g (1½ oz) chickweed
50 g (2 oz) Cheddar cheese
30 ml (2 tablespoons) olive oil
15 ml (1 tablespoon) cider vinegar
15 ml (1 tablespoon) Worcestershire sauce
4 tomatoes

Finely chop the chickweed. Put it into a bowl. Finely grate the cheese and mix it with the chickweed. Beat the oil, vinegar and Worcester-shire sauce together and fold them into the salad. Divide the salad between four small plates and garnish them with tomato wedges. Serves 4.

Chickweed and Almond Gratin

Serve this as a main meal.

350 g (12 oz) chickweed
125 g (4 oz) almonds
40 g (1½ oz) butter
45 ml (3 tablespoons) wholewheat flour
450 ml (¾ pint) milk
225 g (8 oz) Cheddar or Gruyere cheese, grated
freshly grated nutmeg

Heat the oven to Reg 6/200C/400F. Wash and chop the chickweed. Blanch and split the almonds. Boil the chickweed in a small amount of water for 5 minutes. Drain it well and put it into the bottom of an ovenproof dish. Melt the butter in a saucepan on a moderate heat. Stir in the flour and cook it for ½ minute. Stir in the milk and stir until the sauce is thick and bubbling. Take the pan from the heat and beat in all the cheese. Cover the chick-weed with the cheese sauce and grate over a little nutmeg. Scatter the pieces of almonds over the top. Bake the gratin for 20 minutes or until the top is golden brown. Serves 4.

Chickweed and Marmite Sandwiches

50 g (2 oz) chickweed
225 g (8 oz) curd cheese
10 ml (2 teaspoons) yeast extract
12 slices wholewheat bread

Finely chop the chickweed. Beat the cheese with the marmite and mix in the chickweed. There is no need to butter the bread. Spread the filling on six of the slices. Press the other slices on top and cut the sandwiches into squares or triangles.

Chickweed and Potato Soufflé

You can serve this soufflé as a side dish to replace the potatoes, or it could make a light lunch or supper dish accompanied only by a salad.

900 g (2 lbs) potatoes
1 small onion, thinly sliced
125 g (4 oz) chickweed
sea salt and freshly ground black pepper
90 ml (6 tablespoons) milk
2 eggs, separated
butter for greasing

Heat the oven to Reg 6/200C/400F. Boil the potatoes, unpeeled, with the onion until they are soft. Drain and skin them and reserve the onion. Chop the chickweed. Bring 7.5 cm (3 inches) of water to the boil in a small saucepan. Put in the chickweed and simmer it for 2 minutes. Drain it. Put the potatoes, onion and chickweed together through a vegetable mill or rub them through a coarse sieve. Beat in the seasonings, butter, milk and egg yolks. Stiffly whip the egg whites and fold them into the potatoes. Pile the mixture into a deep, buttered, ovenproof dish and put it into the oven for 35 minutes so you have a light, risen soufflé with a crispy golden brown top. Serves 4–6.

Cream of Chickweed Soup

450 g (1 lb) chickweed
2 medium onions
575 ml (1 pint) stock
bouquet garni
sea salt and freshly ground black pepper
25 g (1 oz) butter
30 ml (2 tablespoons) wholewheat flour
275 ml (½ pint) milk
¼ nutmeg, grated
30 ml (2 tablespoons) chopped parsley
50 g (2 oz) Cheddar cheese, grated (optional)

Finely chop the chickweed and thinly slice the onions. Bring the stock to the boil. Put in the chickweed, onions and bouquet garni. Season, cover and simmer for 15 minutes. Remove the bouquet garni and work the rest in a blender to a thin, green purée. Melt the butter in a saucepan on a low heat. Stir in the flour and cook it for ½ minute. Stir in the milk and keep stirring until you have a thick, bubbling sauce. Stir in the chickweed purée and the parsley and bring the soup to the boil. Simmer it for 5 minutes, stirring occasionally. Pour the soup into individual soup bowls and either serve it plain or top each bowlful with a pile of grated cheese. Serves 4.

Medicinal

Chickweed is cooling and soothing for many ailments.

For sores, inflammation and itching: Bring 50 g (2 oz) chickweed to the boil in 1 litre (1¾ pints) water. Take it from the heat and let it stand for 15 minutes. Strain and add the liquid to the water for a warm bath. After the bath, spread the infected parts with chickweed salve.

Chickweed Salve

225 g (8 oz) chickweed, chopped
175 g (6 oz) petroleum jelly
25 g (1 oz) beeswax

Put the petroleum jelly and beeswax into a small casserole and melt them together over a low heat, without letting them boil. Mix in the chickweed, still on a low heat. Cover the casserole and put it into a low oven (70C/200F/Gas under ¼) for 4 hours. Strain the salve through muslin or a nylon sieve into a clean jar. Work quickly as it rapidly starts to cool and thicken. Let it cool so that it becomes firm and cover it.

For tired eyes: Infuse 15 g (½ oz) each chickweed and rose leaves in 575 ml (1 pint) boiling water for 15 minutes. Strain. Dip two pads of cotton wool into the liquid, squeeze them out a little and lay down for 15 minutes with the pads over your eyes.

For constipation: Boil 15 g (½ oz) chopped fresh chickweed in 1 litre (1¾ pints) water until the liquid is reduced by half. Take 1 tea cup full, warm, every three hours.

Veterinary

Give cage birds chickweed to eat and they will thrive.
Hutch rabbits will keep healthy if chickweed is included in their diet.
Weak piglets that are scouring should have chickweed added to their mash to provide them with additional iron.

COLTSFOOT

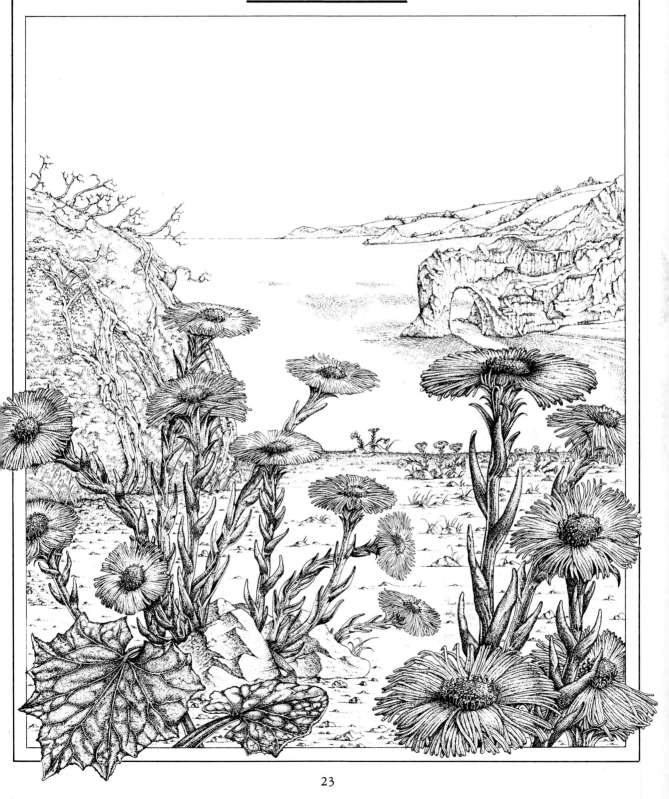

TUSSILAGO FARFARA
Local names: Ass's Foot, Baccy Plant, British Tobacco,
Bull's Foot, Butter, Calve's Foot, Clatterclogs, Cleat,
Coughwort, Cow-Heave, Dishilago, Dove-Dock, Dummy Leaf,
Field Hove, Flower Velure, Foal's Foot, Son-Afore-the-Father,
Sweep's Brushes, Yellow Stars, Yellow Trumpets.

Availability

Coltsfoot grows all over Britain and Europe. In the United States it is found mainly in the North Eastern States. It is not found wild in Australia, but is available dried, and at some herb nurseries. It grows well on poor, stiff soils but flourishes equally in the wet or dry. It can be found by streams, rivers and ditches, on mountainsides, on the edges of woodland and on roadside verges. It often flourishes on railway banks and waste places. The root of coltsfoot spreads widely and so the plants may cover fairly large patches of ground.

The flowers of coltsfoot appear before the leaves, in late February and March (August and September in Australasia). Cut only the heads or the heads and stems with scissors. The large leaves can be picked from April to July (October to January in Australasia).

Both flowers and leaves contain the same properties. Use them fresh or dry them for autumn and winter use.

Coltsfoot Griddle Cakes

Coltsfoot flowers give cakes a sweet and pungent flavour. You can add the petals to basic sponge mixtures or make these traditional farmhouse griddle cakes.

225 g (8 oz) wholewheat flour
2.5 ml (½ teaspoon) baking powder
40 g (1½ oz) butter
petals from 25 g (1 oz) coltsfoot flowers
50 g (2 oz) currants
30 ml (2 tablespoons) honey
125 ml (4 fl oz) coltsfoot or dandelion or another light
   flower wine, or a white grape wine
little butter for greasing

Put the flour into a bowl with the baking powder and rub in the butter. With your fingers, toss in the coltsfoot petals and currants. Make a well in the centre, put in the honey and pour in the wine. Mix everything to a dough. Divide the dough into eight portions and make each one into a round, flat cake about 1 cm (⅜ inch) thick. Lightly grease a griddle and get it hot on the stove. Once it is hot and sizzling, turn the heat to low. Put on the cakes and cook them for about 4 minutes on each side so they are golden brown and cooked through. They are best eaten hot and need no accompaniment.

Coltsfoot Ice Cream

275 ml (½ pint) thick cream
275 ml (½ pint) natural yoghurt
60 ml (4 tablespoons) honey
1.5 ml (¼ teaspoon) fine sea salt
petals from 25 g (1 oz) coltsfoot flowers

Whip the cream until it is slightly thickened. Whip in the yoghurt so the mixture becomes light and fluffy. Whip in the honey and salt and fold in the coltsfoot petals. Put the mixture into a bowl or freezing tray and put it into the coldest part of the freezer or the freezing compartment of the refrigerator (at the lowest setting). Freeze it until it is slushy. Take the mixture out and whip it again so it becomes fluffy and smooth. Freeze the ice-cream for a further 4 hours. Either take it out, leave it for 45 minutes and serve it immediately; or whip it again and put it into a plastic container for storing. It will keep in the freezing compartment of the refrigerator (back at a normal setting) for up to 2 weeks and in the freezer for three months. Serves 6.

Coltsfoot Wine

2.3 litres (4 pints) coltsfoot flowers, yellow parts only
4.6 litres (1 gallon) boiling water
225 g (8 oz) raisins, minced
1.35 kg (3 lbs) light brown (demerara) sugar
thinly pared rinds and juices 2 oranges and 2 lemons
175 ml (6 fl oz) cold strong tea
yeast nutrient
yeast

Put the flowers into a container and pour on the water. Cover and leave them for 3 days, stirring every day. Put the raisins, sugar and orange and lemon rinds into another container and strain on the liquid from the flowers. Add the tea and yeast nutrient and scatter the yeast on top. Leave to ferment in a warm place for 7 days. Strain the wine into a 4.6 litre (1 gallon) jar and fit a fermentation lock. Rack as the wine clears and bottle when fermentation is complete. Leave for 1 year before opening.

Medicinal

Coltsfoot Cough Syrup

125 g (4 oz) coltsfoot stems
275 ml (½ pint) water
675 g (1½ lbs) dark brown sugar

Cut the stems into 3 cm (1 inch) lengths. Put them into a saucepan with the water and sugar. Set them on a low heat and stir until the sugar dissolves. Bring them to the boil and skim. Boil for about 3o minutes, or until you have a thick syrup. Strain it through muslin and pour it into jars. Cover it while it is still warm.

Eat a spoonful whenever you have an irritating cough. You can also dissolve it in hot water and have it as a soothing drink.

Herbal Tobaccos

Whereas conventional tobaccos do nothing but hinder a lung complaint, mixtures containing coltsfoot are believed to positively help it.

British Herbal Tobacco: Take 15 g (½ oz) each dried buckbean, betony, eyebright, rosemary, thyme, lavender and chamomile and mix them with 100 g (3½ oz) dried coltsfoot leaves. Roll the mixture into cigarette papers like conventional tobacco.

Coltsfoot Smoking Mixture: Find several long, pointed sticks and thread coltsfoot leaves onto them. Hang them up in a warm, dry place until the leaves are yellow-brown, quite stiff and leathery. Take them down and wrap the leaves in damp linen. Leave them for 24 hours. Tear out the mid ribs. Pack them tightly into a box, sprinkling in, as you go, a little rum or brandy or a mixture of four parts water to one of molasses or honey. Press the leaves with a heavy weight for 24 hours. By this time they should be in a block. Take it out and shred it. This can be smoked in a pipe or rolled into cigarettes.

Asthma and other respiratory complaints: Put 25 g (1 oz) coltsfoot leaves into a saucepan with 1.15 litres (2 pints) water. Bring them to the boil and simmer until the liquid measures 575 ml (1 pint). Sweeten the decoction with honey. Drink it frequently, by the teacupful.

Or, strain the hot liquid onto 2 slices of lemon in a jug. Sweeten with honey and cool. Drink one wineglassful 3–4 times a day.

Or, put 40 g (1½ oz) dried leaves or flowers into a saucepan with 1 litre (1¾ pints) water. Let them stand for 5 minutes. Bring them to the boil. Take the pan from the heat and leave for 10 minutes. Strain and sweeten with honey. Drink 3–5 cupfuls per day.

Drinking coltsfoot tea instead of ordinary tea over a period of time can very much help with a serious lung complaint.

To make a patient with a chest complaint breathe easily: Burn dried coltsfoot leaves and flowers in the room.

For headache caused by blocked nose and sinuses: Sniff the dried and finely powdered leaves like snuff.

To remove threadveins on the skin; to cleanse and smooth dry skin and to lessen excessive redness: Soak 8 coltsfoot flowers in cold milk and leave them for 4 hours. Take them out and, without draining, wrap them in muslin. Hold the compress against the affected part.

For inflammations, swellings, weals on the skin, erysipelas: Infuse 15 g (½ oz) each dried coltsfoot, elderflowers and peppermint flowers in 575 ml (1 pint) boiling water for 15 minutes. Strain. Bathe the affected areas with the infusion.

Or, dip a cotton wool pad in the liquid, put it against the affected part and secure it with a bandage.

DANDELION

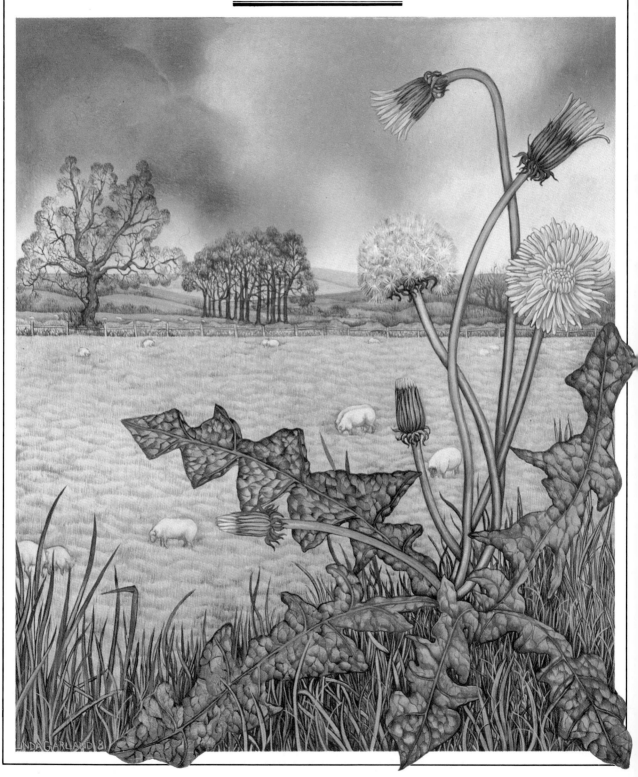

TARAXACUM OFFICINALE
*Local Names: Burning Fire, Canker, Clocks and Watches,
Combs and Hair Pins, Devil's Milk Plant, Dog Posy, Farmer's
Clocks, Four O'Clock, Golden Suns, Heart Fever Grass, Irish
Daisy, Lay-a-Bed, Lion's Teeth, Monk's Head, One O'Clock,
Piss-a-Bed, Puffball, Shit-a-Bed, Stink Davie, Tell-Time,
Woshes, Wild Endive, Witch Gowan, White Endive.*

Availability

The dandelion grows throughout Britain, Europe, the United States and Australasia. It flourishes in open grassy places such as roadside banks and verges, garden lawns and waste ground.

Pick the leaves from February to May (August to November in Australasia) when they are young and tender. Cut them from the plant with scissors and wash them well. Remove the mid ribs if the leaves are very large.

The flowers should be picked when they are not quite fully out.

If you only wish to pick the leaves of dandelions, and are able to watch over some plants, cut off the flower stems as soon as they appear. All the energy of the plant will then be concentrated to the leaves and they will grow thick and keep in peak condition for a longer time.

To gather the seeds of dandelions to sow again or for sprouting in jam jars, collect them towards sunset when the heads are closed. Dry them in the sun, covered with coarse muslin to prevent them blowing away.

The roots of dandelions grown in good garden soil are longer and thicker than those found in poor waste ground. Dig them up when they are two years old. Use a long trowel to avoid breaking them and choose a wet day in October (April in Australasia). Wash the roots thoroughly and cut off the leaves, without cutting into the roots. Dry them with paper towels.

To dry dandelion roots for storing: Keep the smaller ones whole and cut the larger ones, diagonally, into 10 cm (4 inch) long pieces. Lay them on wire racks and dry them in the sun or in an airing cupboard for about 14 days. When dried, they should be hard, brittle and shrivelled, brown outside and white inside. Store them in airtight tins for no longer than a year.

Dandelion Coffee

This stimulates the general metabolism and improves the function of the liver and kidneys, but does not increase heart rate or cause wakefulness. It is an aid to digestion and is good for rheumatism and gout. It can also taste very pleasant and is not dissimilar to ordinary coffee.

Chop freshly dug, washed dandelion roots into thick, diagonal slices. Lay them on a baking tray and put them into a preheated Reg 6/200C/400F oven until they are a good dark brown (about 30 minutes). Cool them and grind them in a coffee grinder so they look like medium ground coffee. Spread them out on the baking tray and put them into a preheated Reg 6/180C/350F oven for 7 minutes.

Dandelion coffee is not very effective if used in a coffee filter or drip pot. For the best tasting brew, put 90 ml (6 tablespoons) dandelion coffee into a saucepan with 850 ml (1½ pints) water. Bring them to the boil and simmer gently for 10 minutes. Strain the coffee into a warm jug and serve black or with milk and cream. Dandelion coffee is not as bitter as real coffee and so you may not need so much sugar as usual.

Mixed Dandelion and Peanut Salad

25 g (1 oz) dandelion leaves
125 g (4 oz) mushrooms
50 g (2 oz) alfalfa sprouts
60 ml (4 tablespoons) sunflower oil
30 ml (2 tablespoons) white wine vinegar
15 ml (1 tablespoon) tomato purée
5 ml (1 teaspoon) ground paprika
few drops Tabasco sauce
175 g (6 oz) shelled peanuts

Finely chop the dandelion leaves and thinly slice the mushrooms. Mix them in a bowl with the alfalfa sprouts. Beat together the oil, vinegar, tomato purée, paprika and Tabasco and fold them into the salad. Put the peanuts into a heavy frying pan without any fat or oil. Set them on a moderate heat and toast them, turning them frequently, until they brown. Divide the salad between four individual bowls or plates and scatter the toasted peanuts over the top. Serves 4 as a main course.

Potato and Dandelion Salad

900g (2lbs) small new potatoes
25g (1oz) dandelion leaves
45ml (3 tablespoons) chopped chives
60ml (4 tablespoons) olive oil
30ml (2 tablespoons) cider vinegar
sea salt and freshly ground black pepper

Boil the potatoes in their skins until they are tender. While they are cooking, finely chop the dandelion leaves and mix them in a serving bowl with the rest of the ingredients. Drain the potatoes and while they are still hot, slice them, without peeling, into the dandelion dressing. Gently fold them in so they become well-coated. Either serve the salad immediately or leave it to get completely cold. Serves 4–6.

Dandelion and Salami Salad

Serve this salad with bread and cheese for lunch or supper or as one of a selection of salads for a main meal.

50g (2oz) dandelion leaves
50g (2oz) peppercorn coated salami, thinly sliced
1 large, round lettuce
60ml (4 tablespoons) olive oil
30ml (2 tablespoons) cider vinegar
5ml (1 teaspoon) honey
2.5ml (½ teaspoon) dried mustard powder
1 clove garlic, crushed with a pinch sea salt

Finely chop the dandelion leaves. Cut the salami slices into small squares. Finely shred the lettuce. Mix these together in a salad bowl. Beat the remaining ingredients together to make the dressing and fold them into the salad. Serve immediately so the lettuce stays crisp.

Stir-fried Beef with Dandelions

675g (1½lbs) minced or ground beef
45g (1½oz) dandelion leaves, finely chopped
60ml (4 tablespoons) chopped parsley
2 cloves garlic, chopped

Heat a heavy frying pan on a high heat with no fat. Put in the beef, break it up with a metal spoon and stir it about until the fat begins to run. Put in the dandelions, parsley and garlic and continue stirring until the meat browns. Serve with plainly boiled potatoes or brown rice. Serves 4.

Pork with Dandelion Stuffing

One piece blade of pork weighing, with the bone, around 1kg (2¼lb)
25g (1oz) dandelion leaves
1 medium onion
1 medium cooking apple
25g (1oz) pork dripping or fat
60ml (4 tablespoons) coarse oatmeal
4 sage leaves, chopped
sea salt and freshly ground black pepper

Heat the oven to Reg 4/180C/350F. Bone the pork and open it out. Finely chop the dandelion leaves and the onion. Peel, core and finely chop the apple. Melt the dripping in a frying pan on a low heat. Mix in the onion and apple and cook them until the onion is soft. Stir in the oatmeal and cook it, stirring, for 1 minute, so it begins to swell. Take the pan from the heat and mix in the dandelion leaves and sage. Season well. Lay the stuffing on the cut surface of the pork. Reshape the pork and tie it with fine cotton string. Set it on a rack in a roasting tin and roast it for 1½ hours or until it is done to your liking. Serve the pork plainly, with roast potatoes.

Salt Pork with Dandelions

675–900g (1½–2lbs) salt pork
1 carrot
1 onion
1 stick celery
bouquet garni
50g (2oz) dandelion leaves
30ml (2 tablespoons) chopped savory
15ml (1 tablespoon) light brown (Barbados) sugar
60ml (4 tablespoons) cider vinegar

Boil the pork for 1 hour with the carrot, onion, celery and bouquet garni. Lift it out of the pan, cut off the rind, and pull out the bones. Cut the meat into 2cm (¾ inch) dice. Heat a large, heavy frying pan on a high heat with no fat. Put in the pork and stir it around until it browns. Mix in the dandelions, savory and sugar. Pour in the vinegar and let it bubble. Take the pan from the heat and serve as soon as you can. Potatoes, plainly boiled in their skins, are the best accompaniment. Serves 4.

Pork, Apple and Dandelion Salad

350 g (12 oz) cold roast pork
1 large cooking apple
60 ml (4 tablespoons) chopped dandelion leaves
6 large sage leaves, chopped
45 ml (3 tablespoons) cider vinegar
30 ml (2 tablespoons) sunflower oil
1.5 ml (¼ teaspoon) mustard powder
freshly ground black pepper
pinch sea salt

Cut the pork into 1.5 cm (½ inch) dice. Core the apple and chop it in to pieces the same size. Put the pork, apple, dandelion leaves and sage into a bowl. Beat the remaining ingredients together and fold them into the salad. Serves 4 as a light meal.

Dandelion Beer

225 g (8 oz) dandelion leaves
4.6 litres (1 gallon water)
1 lemon
450 g (1 lb) light brown (demerara) sugar
25 g (1 oz) cream of tartar
15 ml (1 tablespoon) dried yeast
20 ml (4 teaspoons) light brown (demerara) sugar
  for bottling

Put the dandelion leaves into a large pan with the water and the thinly pared rind of the lemon. Bring them to the boil and boil for 10 minutes. Put the sugar and cream of tartar into a large container. Strain in the liquid from the dandelion leaves. Stir until the sugar dissolves, and cool the mixture to blood heat. Add the lemon juice and sprinkle the yeast on top. Cover and leave in a warm place to ferment for 3 days or until fermentation stops. Rack off the beer and bottle it, adding 2.5 ml (½ teaspoon) sugar per 575 ml (1 pint). Leave the beer undisturbed until it is clear (about 1 week).

Dandelion and Ginger Wine

4.6 litres (1 gallon) dandelion heads
4.6 litres (1 gallon) water, boiling
1 orange
1 lemon
15 g (½ oz) root ginger, bruised
225 g (8 oz) raisins, minced
1.8 kg (4 lbs) light brown (demerara) sugar
175 ml (6 fl oz) cold strong tea
yeast
yeast nutrient

Put the flowers into a container and pour on the water. Stir, cover and leave for 3 days, stirring every day. Strain the liquid into a pan and put in the thinly pared rinds of the orange and lemon and the root ginger. Bring to the boil and simmer for 30 minutes. Put the juices of the orange and lemon, the raisins and sugar into a container and strain on the liquid. Add the tea and cool the mixture to blood heat. Add the yeast nutrient and sprinkle the yeast on top. Cover and leave in a warm place to ferment for 7 days. Strain the wine into a 4.6 litre (1 gallon) jar and fit a fermentation lock. Rack as the wine clears and bottle it when fermentation is complete. Leave the wine for 1 year before opening. It should be a clear yellow colour with a slightly pungent flavour.

Medicinal

A liver stimulant and general tonic: Infuse 25 g (1 oz) mixed dandelion, nettle and mistletoe leaves in 575 ml (1 pint) boiling water for 10 minutes. Strain. Sweeten with honey or molasses and drink a wineglassful three times a day.

For gall stones: Put 25 g (1 oz) each dandelion root, parsley root and lemon balm leaves into a saucepan with 15 g (½ oz) licorice root and 2.3 litres (4 pints) water. Bring them to the boil and simmer until the liquid has reduced by half. Strain. Drink 1 wineglassful every 2 hours.

For jaundice in children: Put into a saucepan 25 g (1 oz) dandelion root, 15 g (½ oz) ginger root, 15 g (½ oz) caraway seeds, 15 g (½ oz) cinnamon bark and 7 g (¼ oz) senna leaves. Add 1.6 litres (3 pints) water, bring to the boil and boil until the liquid measures 850 ml (1½ pints). Strain. Dissolve 225 g (8 oz) honey in the liquid and bring it to the boil again. Skim until clear and then cool. Give the syrup frequently in doses of 5 ml (1 teaspoon).

For bilious attacks: Infuse 25 g (1 oz) chopped dandelion leaves in 575 ml (1 pint) boiling water for 10 minutes. Strain and sweeten with honey. Drink 1 wineglassful 3 times a day.

For habitual constipation: Dandelion can be a mild laxative. Boil 15 ml (1 tablespoon) dandelion root in 575 ml (1 pint) water for 15 minutes. Strain. Drink 1 wineglassful three times a day. This also improves digestion.

For scurvy, scrofula, eczema and other eruptions on the skin: Put 50 g (2 oz) dandelion leaves or root into a saucepan with 1.15 litres (2 pints) water. Bring them to the boil and boil until the liquid is reduced to 1 pint. Take 1 wineglassful every three hours.

For rheumatism: Boil 25 g (1 oz) dandelion root in 850 ml (1½ pints) water for 20 minutes. Strain. Drink 1 wineglassful twice a day.
  Also, drinking an infusion of dandelion leaves [25 g (1 oz) to 575 ml (1 pint) boiling water] three times a day will help rheumatic and arthritic joints. Dandelion and agrimony tea, taken over several years will help remove the acid deposits, that are a cause of rheumatism and arthritis, from the body.

For warts: Squeeze the milky juice from the stalk of a dandelion onto the warts and leave it to dry on. Repeat frequently until the warts turn black and disappear.

To beautify the face and remove blemishes and freckles: Pick dandelion flowers just as they are coming into bloom. Boil 25 g (1 oz) flowers in 1 litre (1¾ pints) water for 30 minutes. Strain and cool. Wash the face with this decoction every morning and evening.

Veterinary

Cage birds are fond of dandelion seeds.
Pigs love to eat the whole plant and will grub for the roots.
Dandelion leaves are an excellent food for hutch rabbits, particularly from April to September when they are breeding.

DAISY

Availability

The daisy grows throughout Britain, Europe and the United States, mostly on soil lacking in lime since it manufactures lime as it grows. In Australia, the daisy is mainly found in gardens although some escape into the wild. It thrives in grassy places where the vegetation around it is kept very short, for example by grazing farm animals, rabbits or the family lawn mower. Both flowers and leaves can be picked from spring until autumn.

Daisies are best used as a pretty garnish to salads. The leaves can be chopped and mixed into all green salads. They have a mild, refreshing flavour.

Pineapple topped with Daisies

1 small to medium pineapple
225 g (8 oz) curd cheese
30 ml (2 tablespoons) chopped parsley
1 clove garlic, crushed with a pinch sea salt
32 daisy flowers
16 daisy leaves

Cut the rind and husk from the pineapple. Cut the flesh into 8 slices and cut out the cores. Cut each slice in half. Arrange 4 pieces in an overlapping line on each of 4 small plates. Beat the parsley and garlic into the cheese. Arrange a portion of the cheese down the centre of the pineapple pieces. Press a line of 8 daisy flowers down the centre of the cheese and press 2 daisy leaves at each end. Serve the pineapple as a first course.

Sweet Tomato Salad with Daisies

This can be a side salad or another first course.

30 daisy flowers
50 g (2 oz) currants
60 ml (4 tablespoons) olive oil
30 ml (2 tablespoons) white wine vinegar
1 clove garlic, crushed with a pinch sea salt
freshly ground black pepper
450 g (1 lb) tomatoes

Put the daisy heads and currants into a bowl. Beat the oil, vinegar, garlic and pepper together and stir them into the daisies and currants. Leave them for 20 minutes, which is just long enough for the currants to soak up the dressing, but is short enough for the daisies not to close up. Slice the tomatoes into rounds and arrange them in a flat serving dish. Spoon the dressing, daisies and currants over the top, making sure that the daisies face upwards. Serves 4.

Daisy Leaf and Cucumber Salad

1 medium sized cucumber
25 g (1 oz) daisy leaves
30 ml (2 tablespoons) chopped mint
5 ml (1 teaspoon) dill seeds
60 ml (4 tablespoons) olive oil
30 ml (2 tablespoons) white wine vinegar
1 clove garlic crushed with a pinch sea salt
freshly ground black pepper

Quarter the cucumber lengthways and thinly slice it. Chop the daisy leaves quite coarsely. Put the cucumber and daisy leaves into a bowl with the mint and dill seeds. Beat the remaining ingredients together and fold them into the salad. Serves 4.

Medicinal

To cure blemishes on the skin: Dab them with the juice from a daisy stalk.

For a red nose or blotches on the face: Infuse 30 ml (2 tablespoons) daisy flowers in a teacup of boiling water for 1 hour. Bathe the face with the infusion and leave it to dry naturally. Make the infusion every night at twilight just before the daisy heads close.

For bruises and swellings: Bruise the leaves and lay them on the affected part. Also, drink a cupful of daisy tea made with 15 g flowers to 275 ml (½ oz to ½ pint) boiling water, several times a day.

For skin diseases and such as eczema and scabbing: Put 40 g (1½ oz) fresh leaves and flowers into a saucepan with cold water. Bring them to the boil and simmer them for 2 minutes. Let the decoction stand for 10 minutes. Strain it. Take 1 cupful three times a day between meals.

To heal wounds and counteract the debility that follows injuries: Drink the daisy decoction as above.

For mouth ulcers: Chew the fresh leaves.

To help watery eyes: Infuse 25 g (1 oz) daisy leaves and flowers in 575 ml (1 pint) boiling water until lukewarm. Strain and use as an eyebath.

An ointment for sore eyes

50 g (2 oz) daisy leaves and flowers, chopped
200 g (7 oz) petroleum jelly
25 g (1 oz) beeswax

Put the petroleum jelly and beeswax into a small casserole and melt them together on a low heat. Stir in the daisy flowers. Bring the mixture to just below boiling point. Cover the casserole and put it into a low oven 70C/200F/gas under ¼ for 2 hours. Working quickly so it does not solidify, strain the ointment through muslin or a nylon sieve into a pot. Cover it when it has cooled and set.

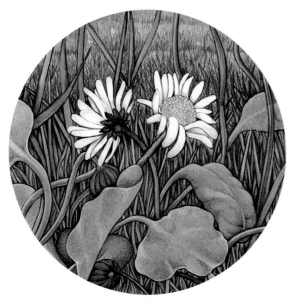

GARLIC MUSTARD

Availability

Garlic Mustard grows throughout the British Isles, in most European countries, and in Scandinavia. In America it is found mostly in the North Eastern and Mid Western States. It is not found wild in Australia.

Garlic Mustard grows mainly along hedge banks and by the edges of woods. Pick the leaves only in spring (March, April and early May in the northern hemisphere). Once the white flowers are fully open, the plants become leggy and the leaves slightly tough. The leaves near the tops of the stems are a brighter green, more tender and have a better flavour than the lower ones. There may be a second crop of young leaves in September if the weather is warm, but these may be difficult to find without the flowers as a guide.

Garlic Mustard Cheese

125 g (4 oz) curd cheese
60 ml (4 tablespoons) chopped garlic mustard leaves
30 ml (2 tablespoons) chopped parsley
30 ml (2 tablespoons) chopped chives
sea salt and freshly ground black pepper

Put the cheese into a bowl, beat in the leaves and herbs and season to taste. Spread the cheese on bread or crackers, eat it with a salad as a main course or, for a first course, pile it on top of tomato slices or rings of fruit such as apple, pineapple or grapefruit. The leaves give a mild and very slightly bitter garlic flavour.

Garlic Mustard Mayonnaise

If you like the flavour of garlic but find a conventional garlic mayonnaise too strong, then you will probably find one made with garlic mustard ideal. Use the youngest, brightest green leaves.

30 ml (2 tablespoons) chopped garlic mustard leaves
1 egg yolk
2.5 ml (½ teaspoon) mustard powder
freshly ground black pepper
125 ml (4 fl oz) olive oil
15-30 ml (1-2 tablespoons) white wine vinegar

Put the mustard leaves, egg yolk, mustard powder and pepper into a bowl and beat them together, either with a wooden spoon or an electric whisk. Beat in, drop by drop, 30 ml (2 tablespoons) of the oil and then 10 ml (2 teaspoons) of the vinegar. Gradually beat in the rest of the oil. Taste the mayonnaise and add more vinegar to your liking.

Use the mayonnaise for coating eggs, all kinds of sea food and also haricot and butter (lima) beans. If you stir it into a mixture of chopped raw cauliflower, celery, cucumber and sweet green peppers you have a tasty and crunchy side salad.

Garlic Mustard Dip

Make the cheese as above and gradually beat in 150 ml (¼ pint) of either soured cream or natural yoghurt. Serve it with small crackers or sticks of raw vegetables such as celery and carrot.

Lamb Chops with Garlic Mustard

4 lamb chops
little butter for greasing
1 small onion, finely chopped
150 ml (¼ pint) dry red wine
60 ml (4 tablespoons) garlic mustard leaves

Lightly butter a heavy frying pan and set it on a high heat. When it is hot, put in the chops and brown them on both sides. Lower the heat and continue to fry them until they are cooked through (about 20 minutes). Pour off all but a thin film of fat from the pan, leaving the chops. Put the pan back on a low heat. Put in the onion and cook until it is soft. Raise the heat, pour in the wine and bring it to the boil. Put in the garlic mustard leaves and cook until the wine has reduced by half. Serve the chops with the sauce spooned over them. The garlic mustard leaves will give the dish a bitter-sharp flavour which is just right for the rich meat. Serves 4 if the chops are large.

Medicinal

To warm the stomach and strengthen the digestive juices: Eat slowly a few leaves on their own.

To excite sneezing: Sniff a few of the seeds up the nostrils.

For gangrene and ulcers: Make a compress of the leaves. Simmer 25 g (1 oz) of the leaves in 225 ml (8 fl oz) water for 10 minutes. Strain. Dip a cotton or gauze pad in the strained liquid and place it on the affected area while it is still warm. Bandage it in place. When the compress cools, reheat the liquid and repeat the process.

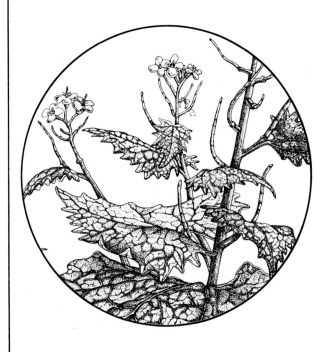

GROUND ELDER

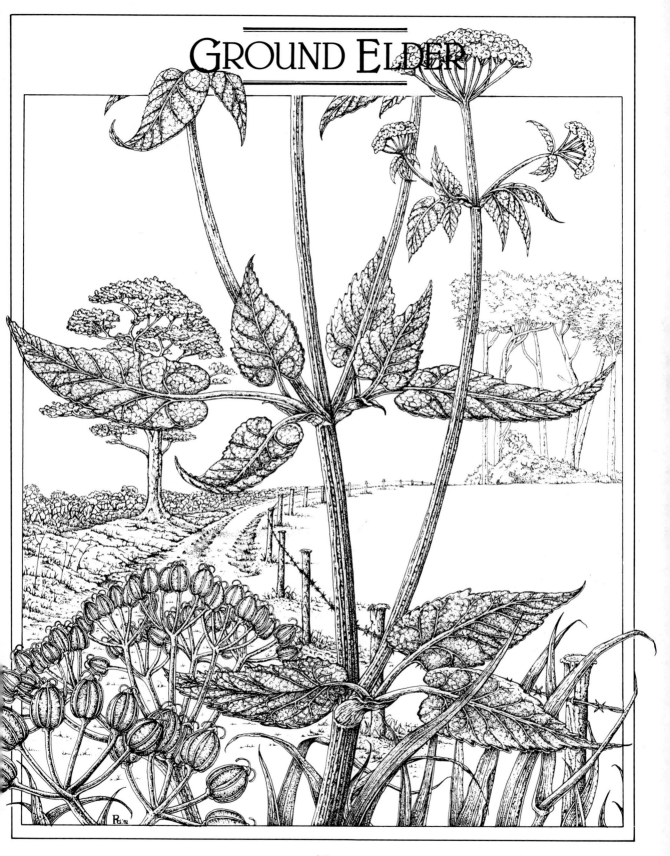

AEGOPODIUM PODAGRARIA

Local Names: Ashweed, Bishop's Elder, Bishop's Weed, Dog Eller, Dutch Elder, Farmer's Plague, Garden Plague, Goat's Foot, Gout Weed, Ground Ash, Pot-Ash, Jack-Jump-About, Kesh, White-Ash, Wild-Elder, Wild Esh.

Availability

Ground Elder grows throughout the British Isles, Scandinavia and Europe and can be found in the Western and Mid Western States of America, but is not found wild in Australia.

It favours damp, shady places and also cultivated farmland and garden plots where it can easily take over and become a nuisance. If you would like to cultivate a patch in the garden that has established itself naturally, try to grow it in a sunken bath, or surround it with sunken bricks as you would mint, to prevent it from spreading.

The young shoots should be picked in spring when they are about 6 inches high (late March and April in the northern hemisphere). After this they become too tough and bitter. Both the leaves and the stems can be used at first but later, check to see if the stems are too tough and if so, discard them.

Chicken, Onion and Ground Elder Soup

The mellow flavour of ground elder when it is cooked makes it a very good plant for adding to thick soups.

1 chicken quarter (or the carcass and giblets of a chicken that you have cut up for a casserole)
1 medium onion, halved but not peeled
2 carrots, roughly chopped
2 sticks celery, roughly chopped
bouquet garni
1 bayleaf
10 ml (2 teaspoons) black peppercorns
2.3 litres (4 pints) water
25 g (1 oz) butter
2 large onions, quartered and thinly sliced
30 ml (2 tablespoons) wholewheat flour
25 g (1 oz) ground elder leaves
sea salt and freshly ground black pepper

Put the chicken quarter, onion, carrots, celery sticks, bouquet garni, bayleaf, peppercorns and water into a saucepan. Bring them to the boil skim and simmer them, uncovered, for 1½ hours, or until the liquid measures around 1.75 litres (3 pints.) Strain the liquid, reserving it and the chicken quarter. (Reserve also the chicken carcass and giblets). Take all the chicken meat from the bones and shred it.

Melt the butter in a large saucepan on a low heat. Mix in the sliced onions and cook them gently, stirring occasionally, until they are golden. Stir in the flour and cook it for 1 minute. Stir in the stock and bring it to the boil. Put in the ground elder leaves and season. Simmer the soup, uncovered, for 15 minutes. Just before serving, stir in the chicken meat. This will make a meal in itself for four people or a first course for six to eight.

Ground Elder and Pork Loaf

25 g (1 oz) ground elder leaves
900 g (2 lbs) pork belly
30 ml (2 tablespoons) tamari (or other soy) sauce
30 ml (2 tablespoons) tomato purée
5 ml (1 teaspoon) black peppercorns, coarsely crushed
1 clove garlic, crushed with a pinch sea salt

Heat the oven to Reg 4/180C/350F. Finely chop the ground elder leaves. Mince the pork. Mix all the ingredients together and press them into a 900 g (2 lb) loaf tin. Bake the loaf for 1 hour so it is firm and the top is browned. Serve it hot or cold. If cold, leave it in the tin until it is completely cold. Serves 4.

Ground Elder Sauce

Serve this with boiled bacon or the Hawthorn Leaf Dumpling on page 66. It is not unlike parsley sauce but has a more subtle flavour, rather like a cross between parsley and asparagus.

25 g (1 oz) ground elder leaves
25 g (1 oz) butter
45 ml (3 tablespoons) wholewheat flour
425 ml (¾ pint) chicken or veal stock
freshly ground black pepper

Finely chop the ground elder leaves. Melt the butter in a saucepan on a moderate heat. Stir in the flour and cook it, stirring, for 1 minute. Pour in all the stock and bring it to the boil, stirring. Season with the pepper and add the ground elder leaves. Simmer the sauce, partially covered, for 15 minutes.

Butter (Lima) Bean Salad with Ground Elder

Raw ground elder leaves have a slightly spicy flavour so they go very well with a spiced salad dressing for a basically bland tasting main ingredient.

These beans can be served as a meal in themselves or instead of potatoes with a cold main dish.

225 g (8 oz) butter (lima) beans
15 g (½ oz) ground elder leaves
150 ml (¼ pint) natural yoghurt
2.5 ml (½ teaspoon) ground coriander
2.5 ml (½ teaspoon) ground cumin
1 clove garlic, crushed with a pinch sea salt
freshly ground black pepper

Soak the beans and simmer them in water for about three hours or until they are soft. Drain them and cool them to lukewarm. Finely chop the ground elder leaves. Beat the yoghurt with the spices, garlic and pepper. Put the beans into a bowl and fold in the ground elder leaves and yoghurt dressing. Leave them to cool completely.

Medicinal

For gout, rheumatic pains and sciatica: Boil 50 g (2 oz) young ground elder leaves in 225 ml (8 fl oz) water for 4 minutes. Drain them and lay them, still hot, between 2 pieces muslin. Lay them on the aching limb.

HOP

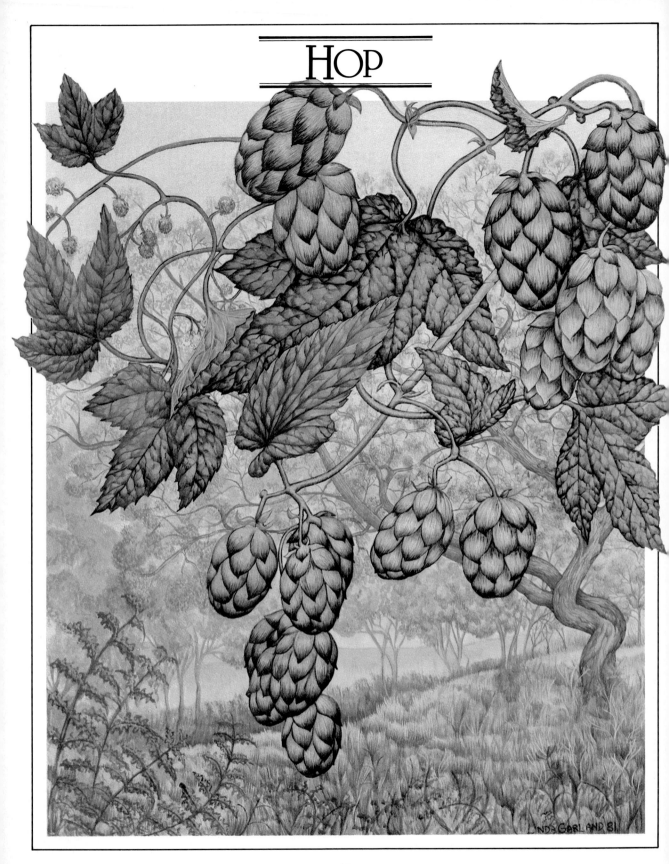

Linda Garland 81

Availability

The hop grows in the midlands and south of the British Isles and in the lowland areas of Europe. In America it can be found mainly in the western and south western states. It is not found wild in Australia but is easy to obtain in dried form. You will find hops twining round hedges and thickets, particularly in damp places. They will probably be most abundant in areas where they are grown for the brewer.

Pick the small, red-tinged shoots in mid-spring (March to April in the northern hemisphere), when they are young and tender and look like asparagus. Break or cut them off to a length of about 8 cm (3 inches). The green, papery textured flowers are ready for picking during early autumn.

Buttered Hop Tops

225 g (8 oz) hop tops
40 g (1½ oz) butter

Melt the butter in a saucepan on a low heat. Carefully mix in the hop tops. Cover them and cook them gently for 10 minutes. Serve them as a garnish for chicken.

Buttered Hop Tops with Lemon

Cook as above, adding a squeeze of lemon juice and some freshly ground black pepper to the pan for the last 2 minutes of cooking time.

Buttered Hop Tops with Cheese

Serve this as a first course.

225 g (8 oz) hop tops
40 g (1½ oz) butter
75 g (3 oz) Cheddar cheese, finely grated
60 ml (2 tablespoons) chopped parsley

Cook as for buttered hop tops. Put a bed of the grated cheese on each of 4 small plates. Arrange the hop tops on the cheese and scatter the parsley over the top. Serves 4.

Cauliflower with Hop Top Sauce

1 large cauliflower
125 g (4 oz) hop tops
50 g (2 oz) butter
juice 1 lemon
60 ml (2 tablespoons) chopped parsley
freshly ground black pepper

Steam the cauliflower whole for 20 minutes so it is just tender. Cook the hop tops in half the butter for 10 minutes, as above. Add the rest of the butter, in small pieces. When it has melted, add the lemon juice, parsley and pepper. Let the sauce come to simmering point. Put the whole cooked cauliflower into a warm deep dish and spoon the sauce over the top. Serves 4.

To dry hop flowers:

Hang them up in branches in a warm airing cupboard until they are pale brown. Store them in airtight tins or boxes.

Baking powder substitute:

Grind dried hop flowers to a powder. Use 15 ml (1 tablespoon) per 450 g (1 lb) plain flour.

Hop Top Scramble

225 g (8 oz) hop tops (or any amount up to this if you can only pick a few)
225 g (8 oz) button mushrooms
8 eggs
50 g (2 oz) butter

Cut the hop tops into 2.5 cm (1 inch) lengths and simmer them in lightly salted water for 5 minutes. Drain them. Thinly slice the mushrooms, and beat the eggs. Melt the butter in a saucepan on a low heat. Put in the mushrooms and cook them for 2 minutes. Add the hop tops and cook for 1 minute more. Carefully stir in the eggs and keep stirring until they set to a soft scramble. Serve either on toast or with jacket potatoes. Serves 4.

Hop Top Tart

shortcrust pastry made with 225 g (8 oz) wholewheat flour
225 g–450 g (8 oz to 1 lb) hop tops (depending on how many you can pick)
175 g (6 oz) cooked ham
125 g (4 oz) curd cheese
4 spring onions (scallions), finely chopped
60 ml (4 tablespoons) chopped parsley
freshly ground black pepper

Heat the oven to Reg 6/200C/400F. Make the pastry and chill it. Cut the hop tops into 2.5 cm (1 inch) lengths and cook them in lightly salted simmering water for 10 minutes. Drain them. Finely chop the ham. Put the curd cheese into a bowl. Beat the eggs together and gradually beat them into the cheese. Stir in the spring onions (scallions) and parsley and season with the pepper.

Roll out the pastry and use it to line a 25 cm (10 inch) diameter tart tin. Put the hop tops and ham in the base of the tart and pour in the egg mixture, making sure it is evenly distributed. Bake the tart for 35 minutes so the pastry is browned and the filling golden and risen. Serve the tart hot or cold. Serves 6.

Bitter Beer

15 g (½ oz) dried hop flowers
450 g (1 lb) malt extract
450 g (1 lb) light brown (demerara) sugar
water
15 ml (1 tablespoon) dried yeast
20 ml (4 teaspoons) brown sugar for bottling

Boil the hops, malt extract and sugar in 4.6 litres (1 gallon) water for 1 hour. At the end add extra warm water to bring the volume back to 4.6 litres (1 gallon). Strain the liquid through muslin into a container. Cool it to blood heat and sprinkle the yeast on top. Cover the beer and leave it to ferment in a warm place for 3 days or until fermentation is complete. Rack off the beer and bottle it adding 2.5 ml (½ teaspoon) sugar to every 575 ml (1 pint). Seal the bottles tightly and do not open them until all the sediment has sunk to the bottom (about 1 week).

Stout

40 g (1½ oz) dried hop flowers
125 g (4 oz) black malt grains
450 g (1 lb) light brown (demerara) sugar
4.6 litres (1 gallon) water
450 g (1 lb) malt extract
15 ml (1 tablespoon) dried yeast
20 ml (4 teaspoons) brown sugar for bottling

Boil the hops, malt grains and sugar in the water for 30 minutes. Strain the liquid into a container and stir in the malt extract. Cool the liquid to blood heat and sprinkle the yeast on top. Cover it and leave it in a warm place for three days or until fermentation is complete. Rack off the stout and bottle it adding 2.5 ml (½ teaspoon) brown sugar per 575 ml (1 pint). Leave it for at least three weeks before opening.

Medicinal

For nervousness, hysteria, delirium and insomnia: Infuse 15 g (½ oz) dried hop flowers in 275 ml (½ pint) boiling water for 10 minutes. Strain and sweeten with honey and drink the whole amount, hot, at bedtime.

For insomnia: Sleep with your head on a pillow of dried hop flowers. This will also help diseases of the chest and throat.

A good general tonic for adolescents to purify the blood: Infuse 15 g (½ oz) dried hop flowers in 1 litre (1¾ pints) boiling water for 15 minutes. Strain. Sweeten if liked, with honey or molasses. Drink a glassful three times a day before meals.

To stimulate the appetite: To 1 bottle of sherry add 45 g (1½ oz) dried hop flowers. Leave to macerate for 24 hours. Strain. This can be taken as it is in a sherry glass or diluted with hot water before the main meal of the day.

For slow and difficult digestion: Take one cupful of the above infusion three times a day after meals.

To stimulate a sluggish liver: Put 125 g (4 oz) hop leaves and shoots into a saucepan. Pour on 575 ml (1 pint) boiling water and simmer for 10 minutes. Strain and sweeten with honey. Drink half in the morning and half in the evening.

For painful swelling, bruises and boils: Infuse 15 g (½ oz) each dried hop flowers, poppy heads and chamomile flowers in 575 ml (1 pint) boiling water for 15 minutes. Strain. Bathe the affected part.

For neuralgia and rheumatic pains: Simmer 15 g (1½ oz) each dried hop flowers, poppy heads and chamomile flowers in 225 ml (8 fl oz) water for 4 minutes. Strain. Dip a large cotton wool pad into the liquid and apply it as a compress.

NETTLE

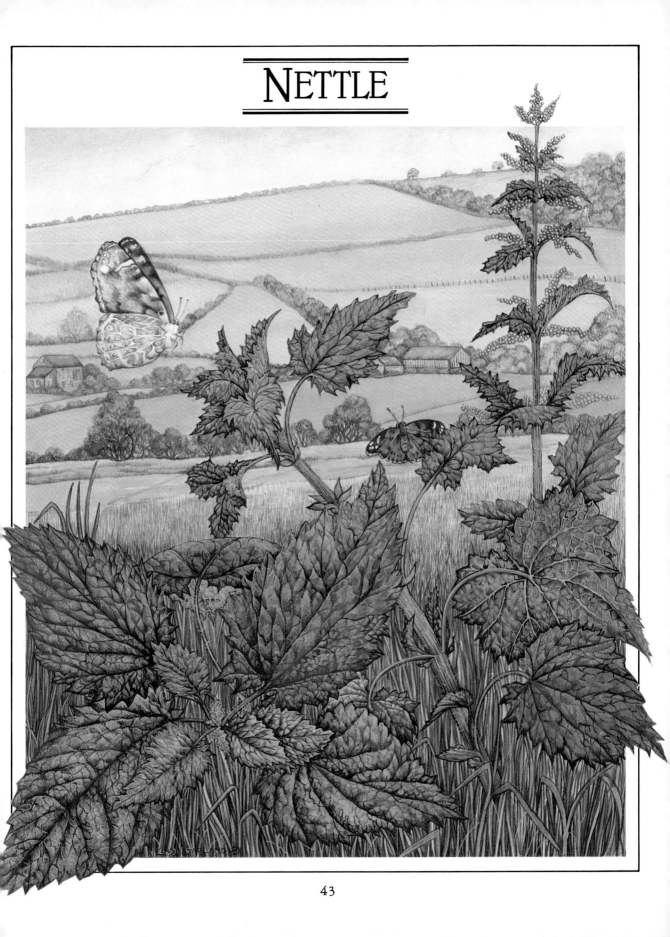

Availability

The nettle is widespread throughout Britain, Scandinavia, Europe, the United States and Australasia. It grows along hedge banks, in woodlands, in gardens, by roadsides and on waste ground and is the commonest of all edible wild plants.

In early spring (March to April in the northern hemisphere), the whole shoots can be picked when they are 8–10 cm (3–4 inches) high. In late spring pick only the tops and young leaves. After the beginning of summer, nettles, although excellent for the compost heap, should not be picked for consumption since they become coarse and bitter and slightly laxative.

Wear rubber gloves when collecting nettles and wash the leaves well before use. Don't worry about the sting—it completely disappears when the leaves are cooked.

Spring Soup

225 g (8 oz) young nettles
225 g (8 oz) potatoes
225 g (8 oz) leeks
25 g (1 oz) butter
1.425 litres (2½ pints) chicken stock
sea salt and freshly ground black pepper
12 large sorrel leaves
40 g (1½ oz) watercress
150 ml (¾ pint) thick cream

Wash and chop the nettles. Peel and thinly slice the potatoes. Wash and thinly slice the leeks. Melt the butter in a large saucepan on a low heat. Stir in the potatoes and leeks, cover them and cook them gently for 10 minutes. Stir in the nettles and pour in the stock. Bring it to the boil and season. Cover and simmer for 20 minutes. While the soup is cooking, chop the sorrel and watercress and add them to the pan for the final 2 minutes. Either work the soup in a blender or rub it through a vegetable mill. Return it to the rinsed out pan and stir in the cream. Reheat it gently without boiling. Serves 4 as a main meal with salad and bread; 6 as a first course.

Brotchan Roy (Nettle and Oat Broth)

A lot of nettles were used in Irish country cooking, as is shown by this recipe and the two following.

75 g (3 oz) young nettles
225 g (8 oz) leeks
125 g (4 oz) smoked belly bacon
15 g (½ oz) bacon fat or pork dripping
50 g (2 oz) rolled oats
850 ml (1½ pints) well flavoured stock
60 ml (4 tablespoons) chopped chives
freshly ground black pepper
salt if necessary

Wash and finely chop the nettles and leeks. Finely chop the bacon. Melt the bacon fat or dripping in a saucepan on a moderate heat. Put in the bacon, brown it and remove it. Mix in the rolled oats and stir until they brown. Pour in the stock and bring it to the boil. Put back the bacon and put in the nettles, leeks and chives. Season well with the pepper. Cover and simmer the broth for 45 minutes. Taste before serving and add salt if necessary. It is a thick, tasty soup and should serve 4 as a main meal.

Nettle Champ

Champ, made with potatoes and nettles, can be served as a side dish or as a light meal in itself. In Ireland, it was once served for the children's supper, accompanied by a glass of buttermilk.

675 g (1½ lbs) potatoes
1 small onion, thinly sliced
50 g (2 oz) nettle tops
275 ml (½ pint) milk
50 g (2 oz) butter
freshly ground black pepper

Boil the potatoes, in their skins, with the onion until they are soft. Drain them, let them steam dry and skin them. Return them to the saucepan and mash them with the onion.

While the potatoes are cooking, wash and finely chop the nettles. Put them into a saucepan with the milk and boil them for 10 minutes. The milk will curdle but this does not matter. Put the saucepan of potatoes on a low heat and mix in the nettles and milk. Season with the pepper and stir on a low heat for 2 minutes so the purée dries a little. Put the champ either onto one large plate or four small ones. Make a well in the centre and put in the butter. Serves 4.

St. Patrick's Day Stew

Young nettles, first appearing in the northern hemisphere around St. Patrick's Day (17th March), add goodness and flavour to an Irish Stew.

50 g (2oz) young nettles
675 g (1½lbs) lean lamb (shoulder or leg) cut into 2cm (¾ inch) cubes
900 g (2lbs) potatoes, cut in 2cm (¾ inch) cubes
450 g (1 lb) carrots, halved lengthways if large and sliced
6 sticks celery, chopped
2 large onions, thinly sliced
30 ml (2 tablespoons) chopped parsley
30 ml (2 tablespoons) chopped thyme
10 ml (2 teaspoons) chopped rosemary
salt and freshly ground black pepper
1.15 litres (2 pints) stock
cold water

Wash and finely chop the nettles. Put them into a large saucepan or casserole with the lamb, vegetables and herbs. Mix everything and season well. Pour in the stock and add cold water to just about cover the main ingredients. Set the pan on a high heat and bring everything to the boil. Cover, lower the heat and simmer the stew for 1½ hours. Serve it in deep bowls so everyone gets a share of the by now very well-flavoured stock. Should there be any stock left over, add it to a nettle soup on the following day. Serves 4.

Nettle Beer

675 g (1½lbs) young nettles
15 g (½oz) root ginger, bruised
2 lemons
4.6 litres (1 gallon) water
450 g (1 lb) light brown (demerara) sugar
25 g (1oz) cream of tartar
15 ml (1 tablespoon) dried yeast
20 ml (4 teaspoons) light brown (demerara) sugar

Put the nettle tops into a large pan with the ginger, thinly pared rinds of the lemons and the water. Bring them to the boil and simmer them for 30 minutes. Put the lemon juice, sugar and cream of tartar into a container and strain on the nettle liquid, pressing the nettles down well to extract as much as possible. Stir until the sugar dissolves and cool everything to blood heat. Sprinkle the yeast on top. Cover the beer and leave it to ferment in a warm place for three days, or until fermentation stops. Rack off the beer and bottle it, adding 2.5 ml (½ teaspoon) brown sugar per pint. Seal the bottles tightly and leave them undisturbed until the beer is clear (about a week).

Medicinal

Hair Care: For a hair tonic, simmer 50 g (2oz) nettle tops in 1.15 litres (2 pints) water for 2 hours. Strain and bottle when cold. Well saturate the hair roots with this tonic every night. This will prevent baldness and make the hair soft and glossy. It will also help keep greying hair a good colour.

For sun-bleached hair or hair that is lank after a long illness, rinse the hair after washing with the above tonic, and let it dry naturally.

For dandruff, simmer 50 g (2oz) nettle tops in a mixture of 1 litre (1¾ pints) water and 150 ml (¼ pint) malt vinegar for 10 minutes. Strain and cool and use it as a rinse after washing the hair.

A spring medicine and blood purifier

Nettle Tea: Simmer 25 g (1oz) nettle tops in water for 5 minutes. Strain. Add the juice of ½ lemon and honey to taste.

For a sore throat: Boil 25 g (1oz) nettles in 575 ml (1 pint) water for 5 minutes. Strain and use as a gargle and mouthwash.

For arthritis and rheumatism: Eat nettles regularly and drink nettle tea, making it from dried nettles when fresh ones are not available. Nettle beer can be drunk to the same purpose.

For high blood pressure: Boil 25 g (1oz) chopped nettles in 575 ml (1 pint) water for 5 minutes. Strain and bring the liquid to the boil again. Bottle it and drink a small wineglassful 3–4 times a day.

For minor burns: Bathe with an infusion of fresh leaves [50 g (2oz) leaves to 575 ml (1 pint) water for 15 minutes]. This is cooling and soothing.

For sores and abscesses: Boil 25 g (1oz) chopped nettles in 575 ml (1 pint) water for 10 minutes. Strain. Bathe the affected parts when the decoction is cool.

SORREL

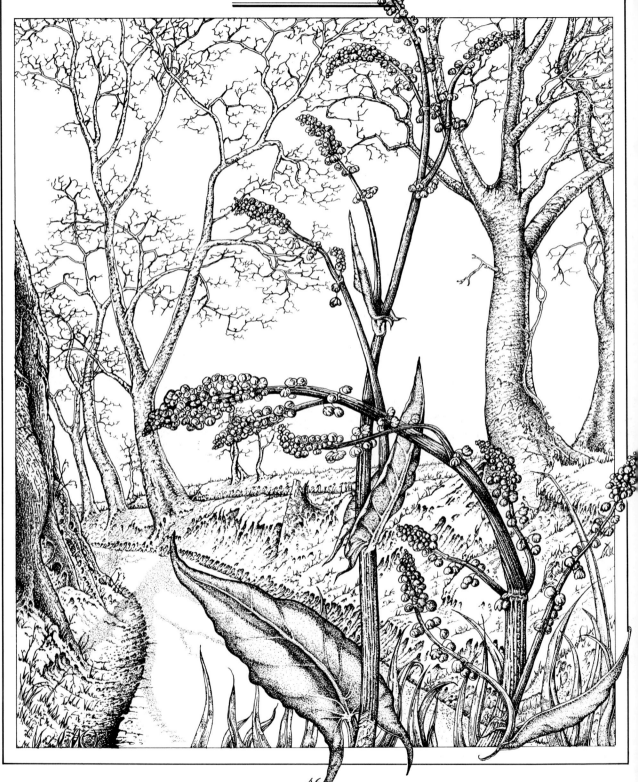

Sheep Sorrel

Local Names: Sourdock, Sour Grass, Sourweed, Red Top.

Common Sorrel

Local Names: Common Field Sorrel, Garden Sorrel, Bread and Cheese, Brown Sugar, Cock Sorrel, Cuckoo's Sorrel, Donkey's Oats, Gypsy's Baccy, Green Sauce, Green Sorrel, Meadow Sorrel, Red Sour Leek, Red Top Sorrel, Sallet, Soldiers, Sorrow, Sour Dock, Sour Grass, Sour Leaves, Sour Sauce, Sour Sops, Sow-Sorrel, Tom Thumb's Thousand Fingers.

Availability

Common Sorrel is widespread in Britain, Scandinavia and Europe and also in the northeastern states of America and in Australasia. It grows best in grassy places where the soil contains iron and can be found in pastures, in clearings and by roadsides. It can also be found in heathy places where there is an acid soil.

Sheep Sorrel, which has smaller leaves but which can be used in the same ways, can be found in similar habitats. It grows throughout Britain, Scandinavia and Europe and is more widespread in the United States and Australasia than common sorrel.

Use only the leaves of both species of sorrel. They can be picked from late February to May (August to November in Australasia). After this the plants will become very leggy and the leaves bitter. To establish a longer supply of leaves, cut off the flower spike as soon as it appears.

Lettuce and Sorrel Salad

1 well-hearted lettuce
20 large sorrel leaves
50 g (2oz) currants
10 ml (2 teaspoons) Dijon mustard
60 ml (4 tablespoons) olive oil
30 ml (2 tablespoons) cider vinegar
1 clove garlic crushed with a pinch sea salt
freshly ground black pepper

Shred the lettuce and chop the sorrel leaves. Put the mustard into a salad bowl and gradually work in first the oil and then the vinegar. Beat in the garlic and pepper. Put in the lettuce, sorrel and currants and turn them in the dressing so they become evenly coated. Serves 4.

Neck of Lamb and Sorrel

Sorrel and red wine vinegar make a contrasting sharp sauce for a rich cut of lamb.

1 kg (2¼ lbs) neck of lamb, chopped into pieces
25 g (1oz) butter
200 ml (7 fl oz) stock
30 ml (2 tablespoons) red wine vinegar
1 clove garlic, crushed without salt
10 sorrel leaves, finely chopped

Heat the oven to Reg 4/180C/350F. Melt the butter in a large, flameproof casserole on a high heat. Put in the pieces of lamb and brown them on both sides (you will probably have to do this in two batches). Remove them and pour away all the fat. Put the casserole back on the heat, pour in the stock and vinegar and bring them to the boil. Add the garlic and replace the lamb. Cover it with the sorrel and put on the lid. Put the casserole into the oven for 1½ hours. Put the lamb onto a warm serving dish and spoon the sorrel and any juices left in the casserole on top. Serves 4.

Sorrel, Mushroom and Bacon Omelette

10 sorrel leaves
1 small onion
2 slices of bacon
50 g (2oz) open mushrooms
6 eggs
30 ml (2 tablespoons) chopped mixed fresh herbs
25 g (1oz) butter

Chop the sorrel leaves, onion and bacon rashers. Thinly slice the mushrooms. Beat the eggs with the herbs. Melt the butter in an omelette pan on a low heat. Put in the onion and bacon and cook them gently until the onion is soft. Raise the heat to moderate and put in the mushrooms and sorrel. Cook them, stirring for 1½ minutes. Heat the grill/broiler to high. Pour the eggs and herbs into the pan and cook, tipping the pan and lifting the edges of the setting omelette with a knife to get as much liquid egg to the sides and base of the pan as possible. When the underside of the omelette is brown, put the pan immediately under the high grill/broiler and cook it until the omelette is golden brown and risen and set through. Either cut the omelette into quarters and serve it hot, or cool it completely (slide out of the pan first), cut it into wedges and take it on a picnic. Serves 4.

Sorrel and Beef Sausages with Sorrel Sauce

675 g (1½ lbs) minced or ground beef
25 g (1 oz) butter
1 medium onion, finely chopped
1 clove garlic, finely chopped
grated rind ½ lemon
¼ nutmeg, grated
12 sorrel leaves, finely chopped
sauce:
25 g (1 oz) butter
1 small onion, finely chopped
15 ml (1 tablespoon) wholewheat flour
275 ml (½ pint) stock
10 sorrel leaves, chopped
6 sage leaves, chopped
juice ½ lemon
pinch grated nutmeg
sea salt and freshly ground black pepper

Put the beef into a mixing bowl. Melt the butter in a frying pan on a low heat. Mix in the onions and garlic and cook them until they are soft. Beat them into the beef, together with the lemon rind, nutmeg and sorrel leaves. Divide the mixture into 12 portions and form them into sausage shapes. Put them into the refrigerator for 30 minutes to set into shape.

Meanwhile, make the sauce. Melt the butter in a saucepan on a low heat. Stir in the onion and cook it until it is very soft and on the point of turning brown. Stir in the flour and cook it for 1 minute. Stir in the stock and bring it to the boil, stirring. Add the sorrel, sage, lemon juice, nutmeg and seasonings. Cover the pan and let the sauce simmer gently for 20 minutes.

To cook the sausages, heat the grill or broiler to high and if you have an open wire rack cover it with foil. Grill the sausages as close to the heat as possible until they are browned all over (about 10 minutes). Serve the sausages and the sauce separately. Serves 4.

WATERCRESS

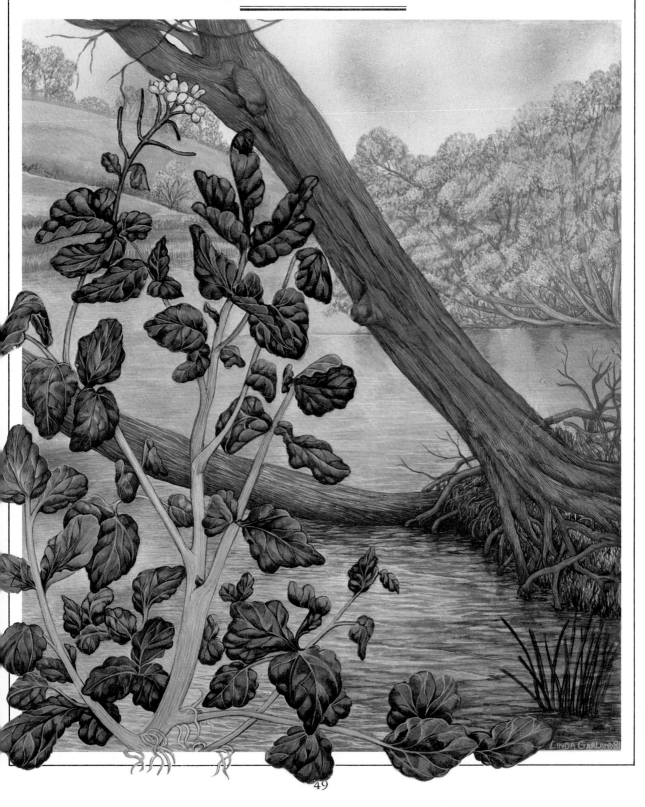

Availability

Watercress can be found throughout the British Isles, Europe, the United States and some areas of Australia. It grows in and by running water and is best when taken from clear limestone springs. Do not pick it from stagnant pools or streams that run through pasture land.

The time to pick watercress is when the leaves are large and dark and the stems thick and fleshy. This will be from spring to early summer, when the flowers appear (March to late May in the northern hemisphere/September to November in Australasia). After watercress has flowered, it goes through another leafy stage and so it can be gathered again in the autumn until the first frosts.

To gather watercress, cut it with scissors or a sharp knife. In cooking and in salads both stems and leaves can be used. You may have to cut off the very bottoms of the stems which bear the rootlets.

Onion and Watercress Soup

225 g (8 oz) onions
25 g (1 oz) butter
10 ml (2 teaspoons) mustard powder
15 ml (1 tablespoon) wholewheat flour
725 ml (1¼ pints) stock
1 bayleaf
150 ml (¼ pint) dry white wine
50 g (2 oz) watercress
1 egg, beaten

Melt the butter in a saucepan on a low heat. Mix in the onions and cook them until they are golden. Stir in the mustard powder and flour and cook them for 1 minute. Stir in the stock and bring it to the boil. Put in the bayleaf and simmer the soup, uncovered, for 15 minutes. Remove the bayleaf. Add the wine and watercress and bring the soup to just below boiling point. Quickly whisk in the beaten egg and carry on whisking until it sets into strands. Serve as soon as possible. Serves 4.

Spring Salad with Bacon

This is a good crisp salad. Have it alone for lunch or as a side-salad with a main meal.

50 g (2 oz) watercress
20 radishes
1 head Cos or Boston lettuce
4 slices lean bacon
30 ml (2 tablespoons) red wine vinegar or malt vinegar
1 clove garlic, crushed without salt

Chop the watercress, slice the radishes and tear the lettuce into small pieces. Mix them in a salad bowl. Dice the bacon, put the pieces into a frying pan and set them on a low heat. Cook them, turning them frequently, until they are brown and there is about 45 ml (3 tablespoons) fat in the pan. Pour in the vinegar and bring it to the boil. Swirl in the garlic and stir in any residue from the bottom of the pan. Spoon the dressing and the bacon pieces over the salad and serve the salad as soon as you can without tossing it. Serves 4.

Potatoes filled with Watercress and Cream

Serve these as an accompaniment to plain meats or alone with a salad.

4 large baking potatoes
45 g (3 oz) watercress
90 ml (6 tablespoons) double cream

Heat the oven to Reg 6/200C/400F. Scrub the potatoes and prick them several times with a fork. Put them on the oven rack and bake them for 1½ hours. Chop the watercress and put it into a saucepan with the cream. Set them on a low heat and bring them to the boil, stirring. Simmer them for 2 minutes. Take the pan from the heat. Cut the potatoes in half lengthways. Scoop out the middles and beat them into the watercress and cream. Pile the mixture back into the potato shells and put them on a heatproof serving plate. Return them to the oven for 10 minutes for the tops to brown. Serves 4.

Trout with Lemon and Watercress

4 trout
65 g (2½ oz) butter
juice 2 lemons
75 g (3 oz) watercress, finely chopped

Clean the trout, but leave the heads on. Van Dyke their tails. Melt 25 g (1 oz) butter and brush the trout with it. Heat the grill to high, lay the trout on the hot rack and grill them for about 3 minutes on each side so they are cooked through and browned. Lay them on a serving dish and keep them warm. Set the grill pan on top of the stove on a moderate heat. Put in the remaining butter and let it melt. Add the lemon juice and watercress and simmer for 2 minutes so the cress wilts slightly. Spoon the cress and lemony butter over the trout. Serves 4.

Medicinal

For anaemia: Watercress is a good source of iron and also of vitamin C, which helps the body to assimilate it. When suffering from anaemia, therefore, eat plenty of watercress salads.

For healthy hair and a clear complexion: Eat watercress regularly throughout its season.

Veterinary

Cows enjoy watercress and it increases the milk yield. Give them two handfuls twice a day.
Watercress is good for a failing appetite in horses, sheep and cattle. Give the above amounts.

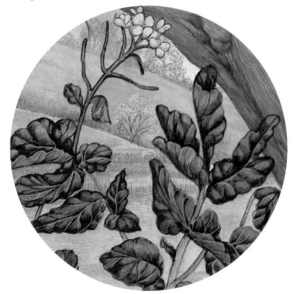

WOODRUFF

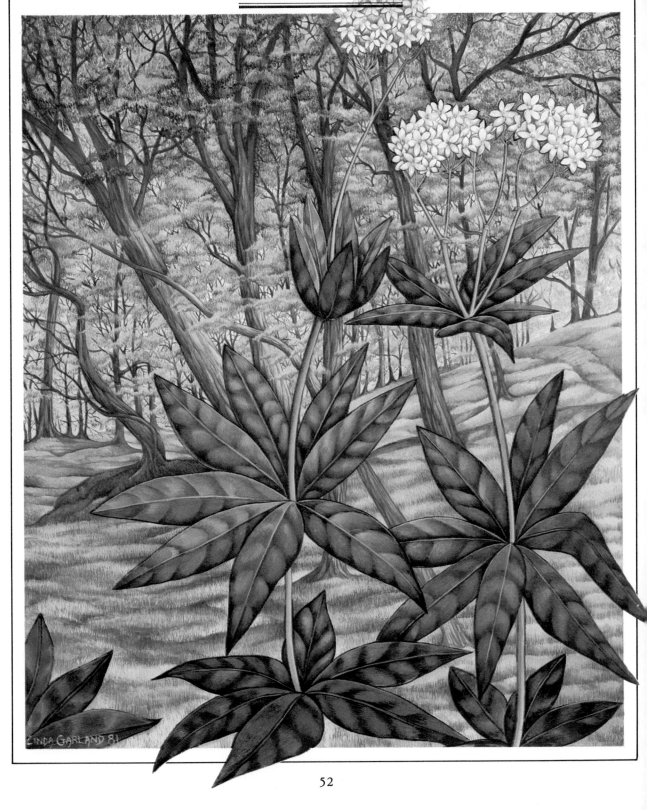

Linda Garland 81

Availability

Woodruff grows throughout Britain, Scandinavia and Europe and tends to favour chalk and limestone areas. It can be found in thick hedgerows and woodlands, especially those containing a number of beech trees. It also grows well in apple orchards. Woodruff likes the shade and will thrive in poor soil. In the United States and Australasia, Woodruff is cultivated in gardens as a rock plant and for ground cover. Some garden escapes can be found in the wild.

Pick woodruff when it is flowering, from late spring to early summer (April to June in the northern hemisphere/October to December in Australasia).

It is best to cut the stems since the fragile roots can easily be damaged if they are roughly picked.

Apple Juice with Woodruff

1 bottle apple juice
4 sprigs woodruff, just in flower

Put the woodruff into the bottle of apple juice. Replace the cap and leave the bottle on a sunny windowsill for one week. Drink it as it is or make the cocktail below.

Woodruff Cocktail

To every 150 ml (¼ pint) woodruff flavoured apple juice add 30 ml (2 tablespoons) brandy. Serve it in small glasses or put it into a jug with chopped apple and crushed ice.

Woodruff and Yoghurt Custard

275 ml (½ pint) natural yoghurt
2 egg yolks
6 sprigs woodruff
15 ml (1 tablespoon) honey

Beat the yoghurt and egg yolks together and put them either into a double saucepan or into a bowl standing on a trivet in a saucepan of water. Set them on a low heat and put in the woodruff and honey. Cover them, stirring occasionally at first and all the time towards the end, until you have a thick, smooth, creamy textured custard. Strain it into a bowl or jug.

You can eat this custard cold or hot and it is superb with soaked dried fruits, stewed fresh fruits, fruit salads and all hot fruit dishes such as pies, crumbles and puddings. You can even use it to top a trifle.

Being made with yoghurt instead of cream it has a very light flavour which is made very distinctive by the nutty vanilla quality of the woodruff.

Sparkling Woodruff Punch

This is a refreshing drink for a hot day. Make up the Woodruff Cocktail and mix it with an equal quantity of sparkling mineral water.

Woodruff Ice Cream

Woodruff gives ice cream and dairy based sauces a nutty, vanilla-like flavour

575 ml (1 pint) thick cream
6 sprigs woodruff
2 egg yolks
30 ml (2 tablespoons) honey

Put the cream into a saucepan with the woodruff. Cover it and set it on a very low heat until it just comes to boiling point. This will take about 15 minutes. Take the pan from the heat and strain the cream. Whisk the egg yolks with the honey until they are frothy, then whisk in the cream in a steady stream. (An electric whisk is the easiest to use.) Whisk the mixture to a light froth. Put it into a freezing tray or bowl and put it into the coldest part of the freezer or into the freezer compartment of the refrigerator (at the coldest setting). Freeze the ice cream to a slush (2-3 hours). Take it out and whisk it again. Freeze it completely. Turn the refrigerator setting back to normal. Take out the ice cream and leave it for 45 minutes. Either serve it immediately or put it into plastic containers for storing. It will keep for up to 2 weeks in the freezing compartment of the refrigerator and three months in the freezer. Serves 6.

Medicinal

To relieve throbbing after a blow on the head: Crush a bunch of woodruff and hold it to the forehead.

To quicken the healing of wounds: Bind on bruised woodruff leaves.

For scabbing: Put 40 g (1½ oz) woodruff leaves into a saucepan with 1 litre (1¾ pints) water. Bring them to the boil and boil for 4 minutes. Cool, strain and bathe the affected parts.

For menstrual pains: Infuse 7 g (¼ oz) bruised woodruff in 100 ml (3½ fl oz) boiling water for 10 minutes. Strain and sweeten to taste with honey. Drink the whole amount 3-4 times a day. This infusion can also be made with 5 ml (1 teaspoon) crushed dried woodruff.

For insomnia, nervous tension, vertigo, neuralgia: Drink the above infusion twice during the day and also on going to bed.

To make sweet washing waters for the face: Infuse 15 g (½ oz) bruised woodruff leaves in 575 ml (1 pint) boiling water until cool. Strain. Wash the face with the infusion and let it dry on.

To "make a man merrie": Steep a sprig of woodruff in a bottle of fruity white wine for 24 hours. Drink the wine before dinner.

Veterinary

To heal wounds and combat ringworm and scabies, finely chop 125 g (4 oz) woodruff, pound it with a pestle and mortar and gently heat it in barely enough water to cover until it is just below boiling point. Measure the volume of the cooked herb and add one quarter its amount in vinegar. Bind this on the affected part.

For failing appetite, give the animal four handfuls of the herb twice a day.

EARLY SUMMER

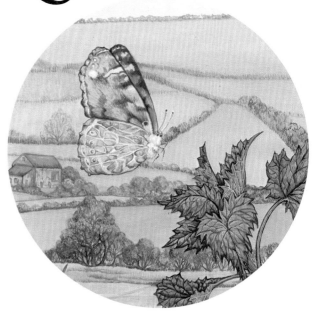

RED AND WHITE CLOVER

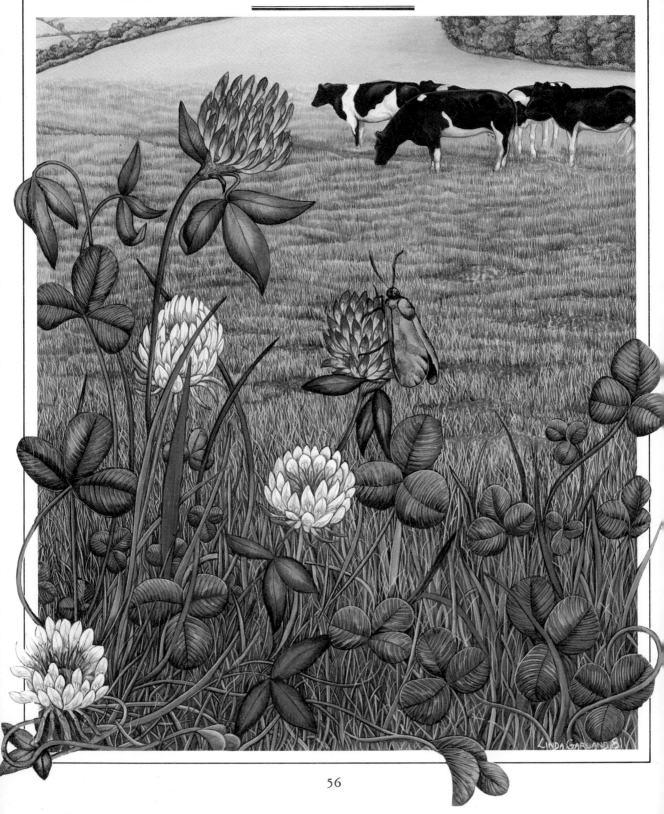

RED: TRIFOLIUM PRATENSE
WHITE: TRIFOLIUM REPENS
*Local Names, Red: Bea-Bread, Broad Clover, Broad
Grass, Cleaver Grass, Clover-Rose, Cow-Grass, Honey-
stalks, Honeysuck, King's Crown, Knap, Ladies' Posies,
Marl-Grass, Red Cushions, Sleeping Maggie, Suck Bottles,
Sugar Bosses, Sugar Plums.
White: Baa-Lambs, Bee Bread, Bobby-Roses, Broad Grass,
Lamb Sucklings, Mull, Pussy Foot, Quillet, Shamrock,
Sucklings, Sucklers, Three-Leaved Grass, White Shamrock,
White Sookies.*

Availability

Both red and white clovers grow throughout Britain, Scandinavia, Europe, the United States and Australasia. You will find them on all kinds of grassy places such as roadside verges, in gardens, on waste places and on the edges of fields. They thrive best on light, sandy soil.

The flowers of both clovers appear very early in the summer and these, together with the leaves, can be picked until early autumn (May to September in the northern hemisphere/November to March in Australasia).

Only pick the youngest flowers. White clover flowers should have all their sections pointing upwards. Once the separate parts start to turn down the flowers are past their best. With red clover, none of the separate sections of the flowers should be drying or turning brown.

Cut off clover heads and sprigs of leaves with scissors and use them as soon as possible for they will soon start to wilt.

Clover Cake

125 g (4 oz) unsalted butter
125 g (4 oz) light brown (demerara) sugar
125 g (4 oz) wholewheat flour
1.5 ml (¼ teaspoon) ground mace
2 eggs, beaten
filling and topping:
125 g (4 oz) light brown (demerara) sugar
125 g (4 oz) unsalted butter
petals from 6 white clover flowers
frosted clover flowers as above

Heat the oven to Reg 4/180C/350F. Beat the butter and sugar to a cream. Mix the flour with the mace and beat it into the butter and sugar, alternately with the eggs. Transfer the mixture to a buttered 18 cm (7 inch) diameter cake tin. Bake the cake for 20 minutes or until it is lightly browned and has shrunk slightly from the sides of the tin. Turn it onto a wire rack to cool.

Work the brown sugar to a fine powder in a blender. Beat the butter to a cream and beat in the sugar. Mix in the clover petals, trying not to crush them too much.

Cut the cake horizontally into two and sandwich it together with half the butter cream. Spread the rest of the butter cream on top and decorate the cake with frosted clover flowers.

Frosted Clover Flowers

Dip clover blossoms first into stiffly beaten egg white and then into icing/confectioner's sugar. Leave them on a rack for 1 hour to dry. Use them to decorate cakes and pretty desserts such as mousses and ice-creams.

Brown icing/confectioner's sugar can be made by putting coarse brown (demerara) sugar, dry into a blender and working it until it is fine.

A Pretty Pickle of Clover

Pickled clover heads keep well. Use them in winter to garnish salads. They also go very well with rich terrines if you lay one or two pickled heads on each slice.

Put alternate layers of red and white clover into jars. Pour in white wine vinegar to cover them. Pour out the vinegar and measure it. To every 150 ml (¼ pint) add 15 ml (1 tablespoon) honey and stir well so it dissolves. Pour the vinegar back into the clover jar and leave the pickle for a week before using.

Clover and Cherry Salad

30 red clover flowers
90 ml (6 tablespoons) olive oil
45 ml (3 tablespoons) red wine vinegar
1 clove garlic, crushed with a pinch sea salt
freshly ground black pepper
125 g (¼ lb) red cherries
1 large, round lettuce

Beat together the oil, vinegar, garlic and pepper. Mix in the clover flowers and leave them for 30 minutes.

Stone the cherries and shred the lettuce. Put the lettuce into a salad bowl and arrange the cherries on top. Spoon the clover dressing over them both to make a pretty summer salad. Serves 4.

Medicinal
Red Clover

Clover and Peppermint Cough Syrup

Take a spoonful of this syrup whenever you need it for the cough that accompanies a cold, bronchitis and asthma.

25 g (1 oz) red clover flowers
25 g (1 oz) peppermint leaves
425 ml (¾ pint) water
225 g (8 oz) honey

Put the clover and peppermint into a saucepan with the water. Bring them to the boil, cover them and simmer them for 30 minutes. Strain the liquid, pressing down hard on the flowers and leaves.

Return the liquid to the cleaned saucepan. Put in the honey and stir it on a low heat until it dissolves. Then boil the syrup for 5 minutes. Cool it a little, pour it into warm jars and cover it tightly.

To soothe the nerves: Infuse 30 ml (2 tablespoons) red clover blossoms in 575 ml (1 pint) just under boiling water for 10 minutes. Strain and sweeten with honey to taste. Drink as needed several times a day. Float a mint leaf on top of the tea if liked.

For a soothing bath: Boil 25g (1 oz) each red clover and chamomile flowers in 1.15 litres (2 pints) water for 15 minutes. Strain and add to the bath water.

White Clover

To cleanse the system and purify the blood: Infuse 30ml (2 tablespoons) white clover blossoms in 575ml (1 pint) just under boiling water for 10 minutes. Strain, sweeten to taste with honey, and drink a cupful three times a day.

A lotion for boils: Infuse 45ml (3 tablespoons) white clover flowers in 575ml (1 pint) just under boiling water for 15 minutes. Strain and bathe the affected part.

Veterinary

Both clovers have been grown as fodder crops, but the white is the most valued in permanent pastures as it provides continuous grazing throughout the year. The red is the one most used for hay and silage.
Both clovers are rich in nectar and loved by bees.
For general debility in cattle, sheep and horses, feed 2 handfuls of either clover twice a day.
For bathing sores, make a strong infusion of white clover flowers.

COMMON COMFREY

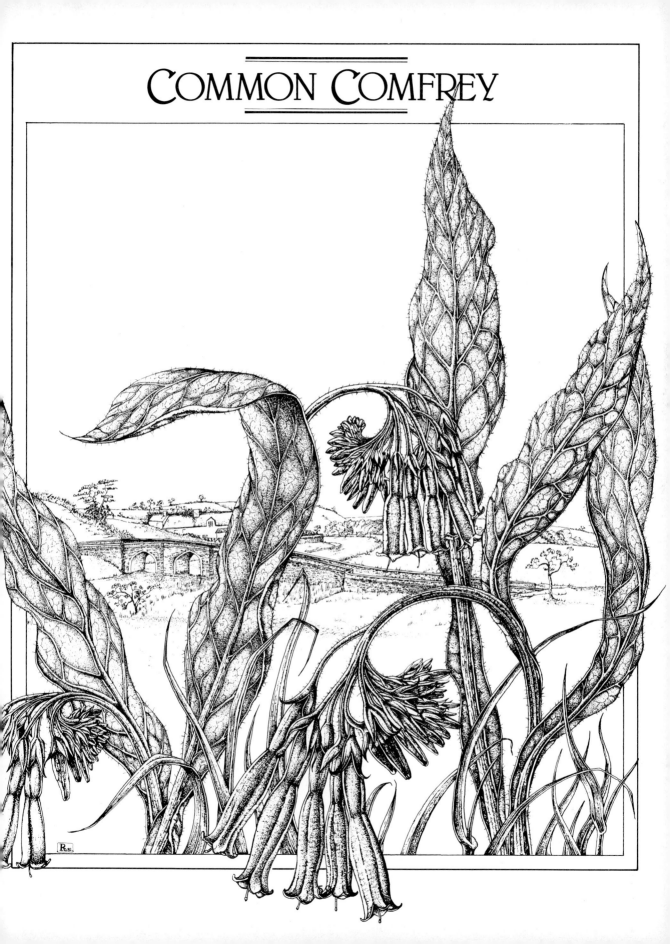

SYMPHITUM OFFICINALE

Local Names: Abraham-Isaac-and-Jacob, Ass Ear, Black-wort, Boneset, Church Bells, Coffee Flowers, Consolida, Consound, Gooseberry Pie, Gum Plant, Knitback, Knitbone, Nip-Bone, Pig-Weed, Slippery Root, Snake, Suckers, Sweet Suckers, Turkey Claw.

Availability

Comfrey grows throughout Europe and Scandinavia and in all parts of Britain, although it is rare in Scotland. In the United States, it can be found mainly in the mid-western and eastern states. In Australasia it can easily be grown in gardens though it is not usually found wild.

Comfrey flourishes best in rich, damp soil that is slightly shaded and can be found along river banks and ditches and in other wet places. However, it also sometimes grows by roadsides and in waste places.

Gather the leaves of comfrey in early summer (May to early July in the northern hemisphere/ November to early December in Australasia). Simply break or cut the leaves from the stems and use them as soon as possible for they wilt quickly. The small prickles will soon disappear when the leaves are cooked.

Lift the roots in early spring. At this time there may be only a few recognisable leaves about so it would be wise to mark the spot of your chosen comfrey plant in the autumn. Dry the roots in a similar way to dandelion roots (page 27).

Comfrey as a Vegetable

For eating comfrey as an accompanying vegetable, pick the leaves when they are small and young.

Boiled Comfrey

Tear 450g (1 lb) comfrey leaves into small pieces. Put them into about 2.5 cm (1 inch) boiling water and cook them gently for 12 minutes. Drain them well.

You can either serve them plainly or pour over them melted butter or equal parts of melted butter and lemon juice.

Comfrey Fritters

For making comfrey fritters, use large, thick leaves. These will give you soft, melting centres inside a crispy batter. A squeeze of lemon juice complements them superbly. Serve them as a stunning first course.

8 comfrey leaves, each about 15 cm (6 inches) long
batter:
125 g (4 oz) wholewheat flour
pinch sea salt
1 egg, separated
15 ml (1 tablespoon) olive oil
225 ml (8 fl oz) beer
sunflower oil for deep frying
1 lemon for serving

Leave about 2.5 cm (1 inch) stalk on the comfrey leaves.

To make the batter, put the flour and salt into a bowl and make a well in the centre. Put in the egg yolk and oil and gradually bring in flour from the sides. Beat in the beer, a little at a time. Leave the batter standing for 30 minutes. Just before cooking, stiffly whip the egg white and fold it into the batter.

Heat deep oil to a temperature of about 180C/350F. Lay the comfrey leaves, one at a time, in the batter, first on one side, then on the other, getting them well coated. Keeping them straight by holding the stalk in one hand and the tip in the other, gently lower the leaves into the oil. Even if the pan is large, it is best to cook only two at a time. Cook the leaves until the underside is a golden brown. Turn them over with a perforated spoon to brown the other side. Lift the leaves onto kitchen paper to drain and cook the rest in the same way.

Serve them, arranged attractively on individual plates, garnished with a quarter wedge of lemon. Serves 4.

Buttered Comfrey

This has a stronger flavour and glossier texture than boiled comfrey.

450 g (1 lb) comfrey leaves
25 g (1 oz) butter
150 ml (¼ pint) water

Tear the comfrey leaves into small pieces. Melt the butter in a saucepan on a high heat. Fold the comfrey leaves into the butter so they become well coated. Pour in the water. Cover the pan and cook the comfrey on a low heat for 15 minutes so it is completely tender and there is no trace of prickliness. Serves 4.

Medicinal

Comfrey Sun Tan Oil

This is a very effective sun tan oil which keeps your skin smooth and glossy. Apply it before you start to sunbathe and reinforce it if your skin becomes dry.

50 g (2 oz) comfrey leaves
275 ml (½ pint) water
30 ml (2 tablespoons) sesame oil
30 ml (2 tablespoons) lanolin

Tear the comfrey leaves into small pieces and put them into a saucepan with the water. Bring them to the boil, cover them and cook them gently for 20 minutes. Strain the liquid, pressing down on the leaves.

Put the sesame oil and lanolin into a small saucepan and stir them on a low heat with a wooden spoon until the lanolin dissolves. Gradually stir in the comfrey decoction.

Put the mixture into a bottle while it is still warm. Put on the lid and shake the bottle well. Keep shaking at frequent intervals until the oil is cool to make sure that the oils and the decoction become well amalgamated. You should end up with something rather like the texture of thin, whipped cream.

Comfrey Hand Lotion

Infuse 25 g (1 oz) chopped comfrey leaves in 150 ml (¼ pint) just under boiling water for 20 minutes. Strain the liquid and mix it with 100 ml (3½ fl oz) glycerine and 90 ml (6 table-spoons) rose water. Stir well and pour the mixture into a jar.

Rub the lotion on your hands after you have been doing rough work outside or if you have had them in water for some time. A little goes a long way.

This lotion is also good for making dry skin on legs and arms soft and smooth.

To sooth a rough, tender skin: Boil 25 g (1 oz) chopped comfrey leaves in 1.15 ml (2 pints) water for 20 minutes. Strain and add to the bath water.

For eczema: Boil 60 ml (4 tablespoons) chopped comfrey root in 500 ml (18 fl oz) water for 5 minutes. Let it stand for 20 minutes. Strain. Moisten a soft cloth in the liquid and apply it as a damp, loose compress. Leave it for 1 hour. Do this three times a day.

To aid in wound healing: Boil 15 g (½ oz) grated comfrey root in 850 ml (1½ pints) water for 20 minutes. Strain. Bathe the wound with the decoction.

Or, grate the fresh root into a bowl lined with muslin. Gather up the sides of the muslin and squeeze out the juice. Use this juice to bathe the wound. It will also quicken the growth and repair of a broken nail.

A cooling and healing poultice for sprains, bruises, swellings, and inflammation: Grate the fresh root into a bowl which is lined with a piece of muslin. Lift the muslin, keeping as much juice as possible. Put another piece of muslin on top and use the wet pad as a poultice.

Or, for the same effect, chop 225 g (8 oz) comfrey leaves and boil them in a very little water for 5 minutes. Put them between two pieces of muslin and use as a poultice.

Or, boil 150 g (2 oz) chopped comfrey leaves in 425 ml (¾ pint) water for 20 minutes. Strain, pressing down well. Dip clean, soft cloths in the decoction and bind them round the affected part.

For coughs, whooping cough and other lung disorders: Put 15 g (½ oz) crushed, dried comfrey root into a saucepan with 275 ml (½ pint) each milk and water. Bring to the boil and simmer for 20 minutes. Strain and cool. The decoction will become slightly jellied. Take it by the spoonful, whenever necessary, to ease coughs.

For diarrhoea and dysentery: Boil 25 g (1 oz) crushed dried root in 1.15 litres (2 pints) water or milk and water for 10 minutes. Strain. Take in wineglassful doses, frequently.

Veterinary

A spring conditioner for horses and cattle: Feed them a handful of cleaned comfrey roots every day.

For sprains and strained muscles: Sandwich a handful of chopped comfrey leaves and a handful of bran between two pieces of flannel and secure well. Boil for 5 minutes. Wring out the flannel and apply it as a hot poultice.

SALAD BURNET

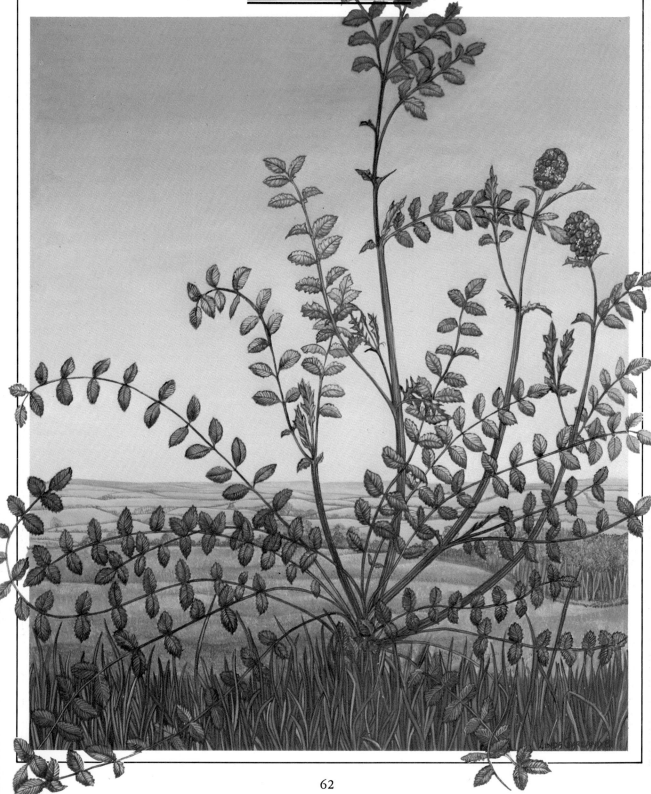

Availability

Salad burnet grows throughout Britain and Europe, particularly in the south. In the United States and Australasia it is found mainly as a cultivated plant, but some escapes can be found.

Salad burnet grows best on chalky soils. It flowers all through the summer but the leaves are best picked in early summer (May and June in the northern hemisphere/November and December in Australasia), before the plants become leggy.

The plants adapt well to being taken into the herb garden. If you are growing them solely for the leaves, cut off the flowering heads as soon as they appear.

When gathering salad burnet, cut off the sprigs of leaves with scissors. When the leaves are very young and soft, the stems can be used in salads and stuffings, but when the plants are older, strip the leaves from the stems.

Lettuce, Carrot and Salad Burnet Salad

Sweet new carrots and a little honey contrast well with the slightly bitter quality of salad burnet leaves.

1 cos type lettuce
225 g (8 oz) new carrots
60 ml (4 tablespoons) chopped salad burnet
60 ml (4 tablespoons) olive oil
30 ml (2 tablespoons) white wine vinegar
5 ml (1 teaspoon) honey
1 clove garlic, crushed with a pinch sea salt
freshly ground black pepper

Shred the lettuce and thinly slice the carrots. Put them into a bowl.

Beat together the oil, vinegar, honey, garlic and pepper and stir in the chopped salad burnet. Fold the dressing into the salad. Serves 4.

Salad Burnet Stuffing

When salad burnet is cooked, it has a slightly honeyed flavour which makes it an excellent accompaniment to pork or duck. This stuffing can be rolled into a joint of pork, put into a bird or baked in a separate dish as an accompaniment.

25 g (1 oz) pork dripping or lard
2 medium onions, thinly sliced
175 g (6 oz) wholewheat breadcrumbs
90 ml (6 tablespoons) chopped young salad burnet
   leaves
4 sage leaves, chopped
125 ml (4 fl oz) dry cider
sea salt and freshly ground black pepper

Melt the dripping in a frying pan. Mix in the onions and cook them until they are soft. Take the pan from the heat and mix in all the remaining ingredients.

To bake the stuffing, put it into an oven proof dish (such as a pie dish) and bake it in a preheated Reg 6/200C/400F oven for 40 minutes so the top browns and crisps.

Burnet Wine

To make burnet wine gather the flower heads when they are just beginning to turn red. Snip them from the stalks with scissors.

2.3 litres (4 pints) salad burnet heads
4.6 litres (1 gallon) boiling water
thinly pared rind and juice 1 lemon
thinly pared rind and juice 1 orange
1.35 kg (3 lbs) light brown (demerara) sugar
225 g (8 oz) sultanas, minced
1 cup strong, cold, black tea
yeast
yeast nutrient

Put the flowers into a large container and pour on the boiling water. Leave them for 3 days, stirring every day.

Strain the liquid into a pan and put in the thinly pared lemon and orange rinds. Bring them to the boil and simmer them for 30 minutes.

Put the juices of the lemon and orange, the raisins and the sugar into a container and strain on the liquid. Add the tea and cool the mixture to blood heat. Add the yeast nutrient and sprinkle the yeast on top. Cover, and leave in a warm place to ferment for 7 days.

Strain the wine into a jar and fit a fermentation lock. Rack as the wine clears and bottle it when fermentation is complete. Leave the wine for at least 6 months before opening.

It is a lovely golden, flower scented wine.

Salad Burnet Lemonade

This is a refreshing, bitter-sweet, honeyed lemonade

30 ml (2 tablespoons) chopped salad burnet leaves
1 lemon
850 ml (1½ pints) boiling water
20 ml (4 teaspoons) honey

Put the salad burnet leaves into a jug. Grate in the lemon rinds. Cut the pith from the lemon and thinly slice the flesh. Put the flesh only into the jug.

Pour on the boiling water. Add the honey and stir for it to dissolve. Leave the drink until it is cold, stir and strain it. Drink it at room temperature or iced.

Medicinal

Veterinary

Salad burnet is an extremely nutritious food for both sheep and cattle and it was often sown as a fodder plant on chalk soils where the grasses were not providing complete cover. It keeps green all the winter, even on dry pastures and has a larger nutritive content than many grasses. When it is full grown, however, cattle do not like it as much as they do clover.

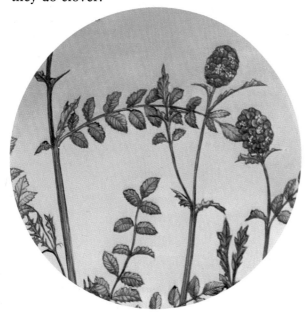

HAWTHORN

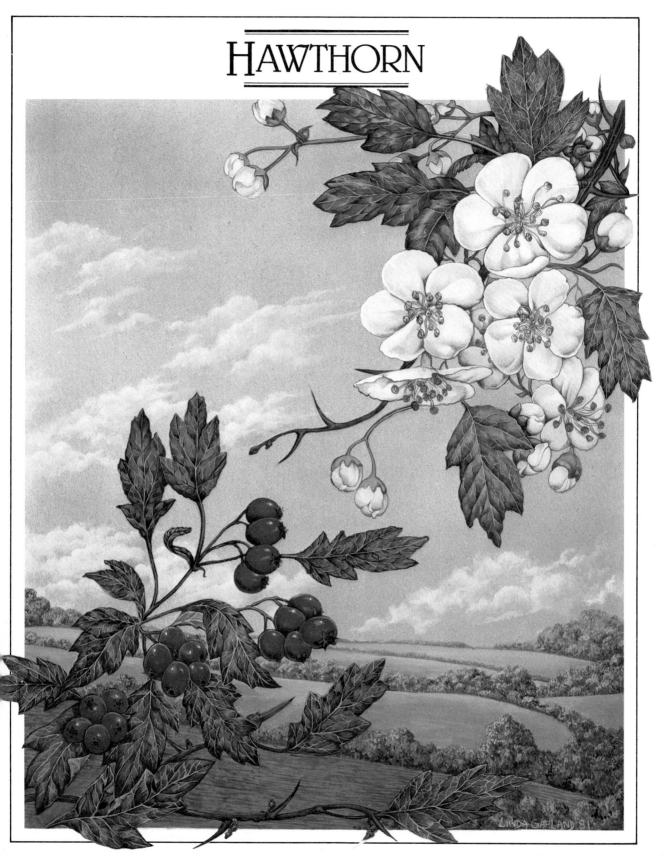

CRATAEGUS MONOGYNA
Local Names: Aglet Tree, Azzy-Tree, Bird Eagles,
Bread-and-Cheese-Tree, Coockoo's-Bread-and-Cheese-Tree,
Hag, Hagbush, Hag-Thorn, Heg-Peg-Bush, Hipperty-Haw,
Holy Innocents, Ladies' Meat, Mayblossom, May Tree,
May-Bush, Moon Flower, Pegall Bush, Quick, Quickthorn,
Scrog-Bush, Whitethorn

Availability

The hawthorn grows throughout Britain and Europe, although it does not occur at all in the north of Scotland. On farmland, it is often cut and woven to make hedges and it can also be found growing to its full height in woods and thickets, on pastureland and on grassy downs.

Crataegus monogyna does not grow in the United States, but there are other species which can be used in the same ways. These include the one-flowered haw (Crataegus uniflora), the May Haw (Crataegus aestivalis), the frosted haw (Crataegus pruinosa), the cockspur haw (Crataegus cruss-galli) and the Scarlet haw (Crataegus pedicellata). All these types are most common in the north and mid eastern states.

The young leaves of hawthorn can be picked in late spring and the blossoms during early summer (throughout May in the northern hemisphere). Pick the leaves from the branches, separately, with your fingers, and use scissors to cut the blossoms directly into a bag or container. Try not to include any stalks with the flowers or these will give a bitter quality to anything that is made with them.

The berries, or haws, will be softer and more mellow if you wait until after the second autumn frost before picking them. However the fruit of the may haw in the southern states of America, ripens in May and June.

Hawthorn Leaf Dumplings

For this recipe, pick hawthorn leaves when they have just unfolded so they are still bright emerald green and very tender.

50 g (2 oz) young hawthorn leaves
225 g (8 oz) wholewheat flour
125 g (4 oz) beef suet, freshly grated
10 ml (2 teaspoons) baking powder
1.5 ml (¼ teaspoon) sea salt
150 ml (¼ pint) cold water
450 g (1 lb) bacon
2 small onions
butter for greasing

Finely chop the hawthorn leaves. Put the flour and suet into a bowl and sprinkle in the baking powder and salt. Mix them to a stiff dough with the water. Divide the dough into two and roll each piece out to an oblong about 6 mm (¼ inch) thick. Scatter the hawthorn leaves over the top.

Finely chop the bacon and onions and arrange them over the hawthorn leaves. Roll up each piece of dough from the narrow side. Wrap each roll in buttered greaseproof paper and then in a pudding cloth (an old tea towel is excellent). Tie the parcels securely with fine cotton string.

Bring a large pan of water to the boil and lower in the puddings. Boil them for 2½ hours, topping up the water with boiling water when necessary.

To serve, lift out the puddings, unwrap them and cut each one in half. A good gravy or parsley or ground elder (page 38) sauce are good accompaniments. Serves 4.

Roast Pheasant with Hawthorn Jelly

Pheasant roasted with hawthorn jelly acquires a browned glossy skin. The sauce provides a contrasting touch of sharpness for the rich meat.

1 large cock pheasant
1 thinly pared strip lemon rind
6 sprigs each parsley, thyme and marjoram
45 ml (3 tablespoons) hawthorn jelly
425 ml (¾ pint) stock, made from the giblets
juice ½ lemon

Heat the oven to Reg 6/200C/400F. Inside the pheasant, put the strip of lemon rind and 1 sprig each of the herbs. Put the pheasant into a roasting tin and cover it completely with the remaining herbs. Cover the tin with foil and put it into the oven for 45 minutes.

Remove the foil and herbs and spread the pheasant with 30 ml (2 tablespoons) hawthorn jelly. Return it to the oven for 15 minutes for the skin to crisp.

Take out the pheasant and keep it warm. Set the roasting tin on top of the stove on a moderate heat. Pour in the stock and add the lemon juice and the remaining hawthorn jelly. Bring them to the boil, stirring in any residue from the bottom of the pan. Simmer the sauce until it is reduced by half.

Joint the pheasant. Put it into a warmed serving dish and pour the sauce over it. Serves 4.

Hawthorn Flower Essence

Use this essence in any sweet dish that calls for a little brandy as a flavouring. See Wild Strawberry Syllabub (page 84).

25 g (1 oz) hawthorn flowers
150 ml (¼ pint) brandy

Pick the flowers without any leaves or stems. Put them into a jar with the brandy, cover them and leave for 1 month.
Strain the essence and bottle it.

Hawthorn Jelly

This is a dark, red-brown jelly with a bitter sweet flavour. Besides being a good accompaniment for lamb and game you can serve it with scones and cream or cream cheese.

1.35 kg (3 lbs) hawthorn berries
675 g (1½ lbs) cooking apples
1.725 litres (3 pints) water
450 g (1 lb) light brown (demerara) sugar
    to every 575 ml (1 pint) juice

Wash the hawthorn berries and remove the stems. Chop the apples, without peeling and coring. Put the berries and apples into a preserving pan with the water. Bring them gently to the boil and simmer them until you have a thick pulp (about 1 hour).
Turn the pulp into a jelly bag and leave it to drip. It may take several hours for all the liquid to come through and you can leave it overnight.
Measure the liquid and return it to the cleaned pan. Stir in the required amount of sugar and stir on a low heat for it to dissolve. Boil until setting point is reached and pour the jelly into warmed jars. Cover it with waxed paper circles and cover completely when cold.
Makes about 675 g (1½ lbs).

May Blossom Cocktail

Make the flowered wine cup and add to it 500 ml (¼ pint) hawthorn essence.

Hawthorn Berry Wine

Hawthorn berries make a deep, red-brown wine with a rich smoky flavour. It will keep for up to ten years.

2.7 kg (6 lbs) hawthorn berries
4.6 litres (1 gallon) boiling water
grated rind and juice 3 lemons
pectolase
1.35 kg (3 lbs) sugar
250 ml (8 fl oz) strong, cold, black tea
yeast
yeast nutrient

Wash the hawthorn berries and remove any stems. Put them into a container and mash them well. Pour the boiling water over them. Add the lemon rind and juice and pectolase and stir. Cover and leave in a warm place to ferment for one week, stirring every day.
Strain the liquid onto a syrup made with the sugar and 575 ml (1 pint) water. Add the cold tea, yeast and yeast nutrient. Put the wine into a 4.6 litre (1 gallon) jar and fit a fermentation lock. Rack as the wine clears and bottle it when fermentation is complete. Keep for one year before opening.

A Fragrant and Refreshing Tea

Infuse 15 ml (1 tablespoon) hawthorn flowers, 15 ml (1 tablespoon) chopped lemon balm leaves and 2 chopped sage leaves in 575 ml (1 pint) boiling water for 10 minutes. Strain and sweeten to taste with honey.

Flowered Wine Cup

Serve this as an aperitif

90 ml (6 tablespoons) hawthorn flowers
4 lemon balm leaves
4 thinly pared strips orange rind
1 bottle dry white wine

Put all the ingredients into a jug, cover them and leave them in a cool place for 24 hours. Strain off the wine and chill it very lightly before serving.

Medicinal

For insomnia: Infuse 5 ml (1 teaspoon) hawthorn blossoms in ¼ litre (8 fl oz) water for 10 minutes. Strain. Drink the whole amount twice a day and again on going to bed.

To draw out splinters: Finely chop a handful of young hawthorn leaves and boil them in water for 2 minutes. Drain them. Put them between two pieces of muslin and lay them on the splinter. Or, pound some berries to a pulp, lay them between muslin and use them in the same way.

For sore throats: Boil 50g (2oz) crushed berries in 1 litre (1¾ pints) water for 10 minutes. Strain, sweeten to taste with honey, and drink a cupful three times a day.

For high blood pressure and circulatory disorders: Infuse 10ml (2 teaspoons) hawthorn blossoms in ¼ litre (8floz) water for 20 minutes. Drink the whole amount two to three times a day for several months.

For diarrhoea and dysentery: Boil 25g (1oz) crushed berries in 1 litre (1¾ pints) water for 10 minutes. Strain and take a wineglassful several times a day.

Veterinary

Feed one handful of the young leaves per day as a tonic to young animals who are being weaned. One handful of the fruits fed to pregnant animals every day will guard against miscarriage.

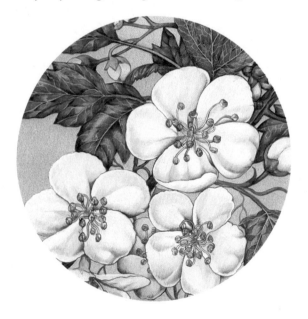

SHAGGY INK CAP

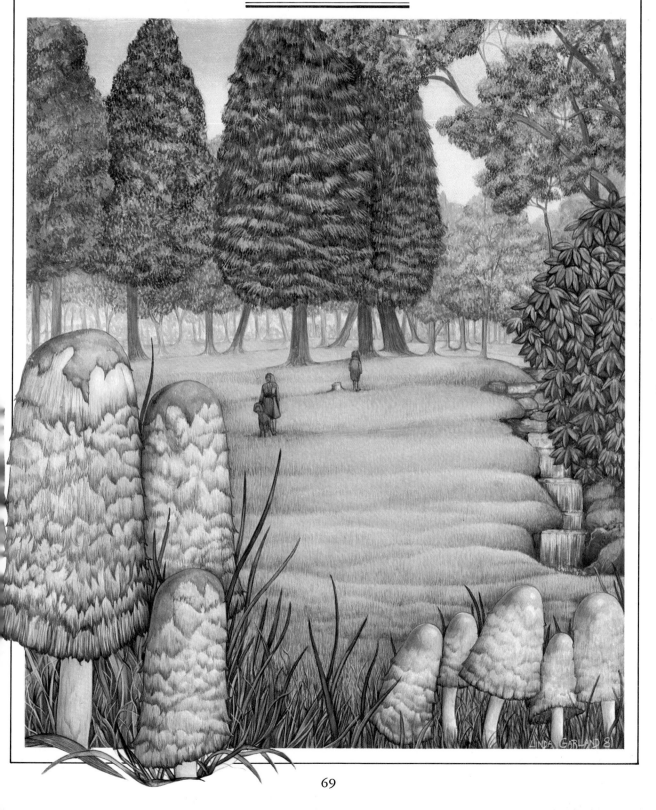

LINDA GARLAND 81

Availability

The shaggy ink cap grows throughout Britain, Scandinavia, Europe and the United States. It grows on short, open grass such as pastureland, gardens, playing fields and road verges. It grows all through the summer months (June to September in the northern hemisphere).

Always make sure that shaggy ink caps are in good condition. When they first grow the gills will be pinky white and the caps standing upright. After a while the gills begin to darken from the edges inwards and the edges begin to turn outwards. When they are too old to use they become damp, and black and start to disintegrate.

Cut shaggy ink caps at the base of the stipe with a sharp knife and carry them home in an open basket. Use them as soon as possible after you get home.

It is not necessary to peel shaggy ink caps before cooking, but make sure that any soil is brushed away.

Mushroom Sauce

This is probably the best way of using shaggy ink caps. It makes the most subtle, mushroomy flavoured sauce imaginable. Serve the sauce with roast chicken, roast lamb or grilled lamb chops, with steak, veal, eggs or white fish.

225 g (8 oz) shaggy ink caps (very young white ones)
40 g (1½ oz) butter
150 ml (¼ pint) milk
¼ nutmeg, grated
freshly ground black pepper
30 ml (2 tablespoons) wholewheat flour
30 ml (2 tablespoons) chopped parsley
grated rind ½ lemon

Cut the caps and stipes of the mushrooms in to 6 mm (¼ inch) thick strips. Melt the butter in a saucepan on a low heat. Fold in the mushrooms and cook them gently for 2 minutes. Pour in the milk and season with the pepper and nutmeg. Bring the milk to simmering point. Cover the pan and simmer the mushrooms for 10 minutes.

Drain the mushrooms, pressing them down well to extract as much liquid as possible. Leave them draining for 10 minutes and press again. You should have about 275 ml (½ pint) liquid.

Put the flour into a bowl and gradually mix in half the liquid. Stir the mixture back into the rest and pour the whole lot into a saucepan. Stir in the lemon rind. Bring the sauce gently to the boil stirring all the time to make it smooth. Simmer it for 1 minute, take it from the heat and stir in the parsley.

Cooking Shaggy Ink Caps

Shaggy ink caps have a delicious, rich mushroom flavour but a rather slimy texture. If you do not mind this quality, serve them as a side vegetable.

Cut the caps lengthways into strips about 6 mm (¼ inch) wide. For every 225 g (8 oz) mushrooms, melt 40 g (1½ oz) butter in a saucepan on a low heat. Fold in the mushrooms and season them with freshly grated black pepper and a little nutmeg. Simmer them gently for 10 minutes.

They can be served as a first course or on toast or as an accompaniment to chicken, veal or egg dishes.

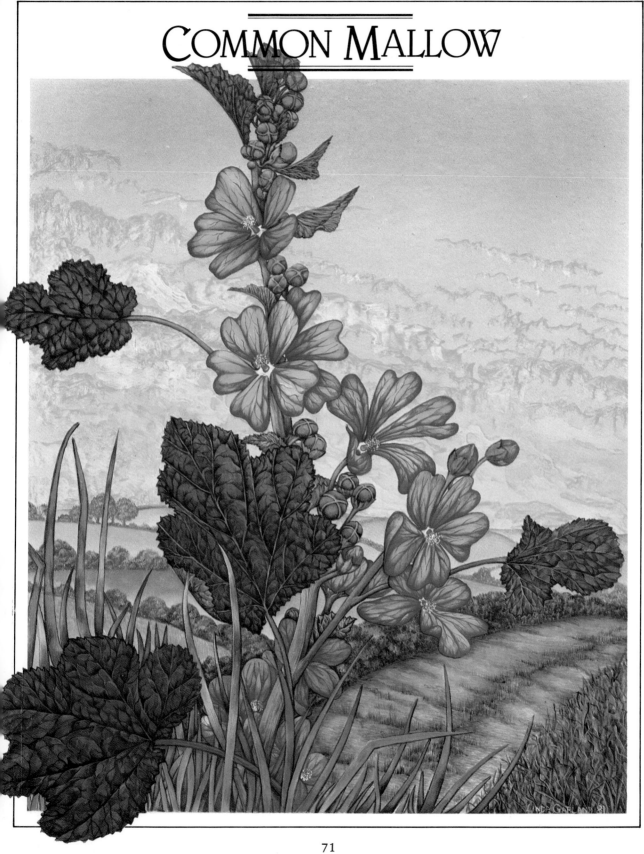

71

Availability

The common mallow grows throughout Britain, Scandinavia and Europe and the northern states of America. It can be found on the edges of fields and by country tracks and lanes, along hedgerows and on waste places and often growing out of the bottom of walls. It thrives near the sea. In Australia *Malva parvifolia* is more common and grows abundantly in both city and country.

Pick mallow leaves in early summer (June in the northern hemisphere/December in Australasia) when they are still pale green, tender and a smooth, almost rubbery texture. Break the leaves from the stems, leaving the rest of the plant still growing. Use them as soon as possible for they very quickly wither.

The tiny, cheese-shaped seeds that appear later in the year are also edible. They are best eaten as a quick and tasty nibble as you go along, since they are rather fiddly to pick in any quantity.

Mallow Gumbo

Mallow leaves, when simmered in stock, have a slight, gelatinous thickening quality, which makes them perfect for using in a gumbo as a substitute for okra.

450 g (1 lb) prawns or shrimps, unshelled weight
675 g (1½ lbs) whiting or haddock fillets
1.725 litres (3 pints) water
1 bayleaf
1 sprig thyme
1 sprig parsley
1 onion, cut in half but not peeled
5 ml (1 teaspoon) black peppercorns
225 g (8 oz) tomatoes
75 g (3 oz) mallow leaves, finely chopped
30 ml (2 tablespoons) white wine vinegar
15 ml (1 tablespoon) tomato purée
10 ml (2 teaspoons) ground paprika
2.5 ml (½ teaspoon) Tabasco sauce
120 ml (8 tablespoons) chopped parsley

Shell the prawns or shrimps and skin the whiting or haddock fillets. Put the shells and skins into a saucepan with the water, bayleaf, thyme, parsley, onion and peppercorns. Bring them to the boil and simmer them for 20 minutes.

While they are cooking, cut the fish fillets into 1 cm (½ inch) strips and scald, skin and chop the tomatoes.

Strain the liquid from the shells and skins and return it to the cleaned pan. Put in the mallow leaves, bring them to the boil, cover and simmer for 15 minutes. Put in the prawns or shrimps, fish, tomatoes, vinegar, tomato purée, Tabasco sauce and chopped parsley. Bring the soup to the boil again, cover and simmer for 5 minutes. Serve the gumbo in deep bowls. Serves 4.

Deep Fried Mallow Leaves

These make one of the prettiest garnishes imaginable, or, if you have enough, you can serve them as an exotic appetiser.

Use only even sixed, unblemished mallow leaves and drop them, about four at a time, into deep, hot sunflower oil, veined side down. They will open flat at first and then gently curl up at the edges; and they will become a deep, transparent green, patterned with veins.

Lift the leaves out with a perforated spoon, very carefully, for they are extremely brittle. Drain them on kitchen paper. Arrange them prettily on a dish, with perhaps a few of the flowers to add to the appearance. Sprinkle them with a very little sea salt and either serve them immediately or allow them to cool. They will still stay crisp.

If using them as a garnish, place the leaves on grilled or sautéed meats or shallow or deep fried fish.

Medicinal

To make a soothing ointment

60 ml (4 tablespoons) olive oil
25 g (1 oz) beeswax
60 ml (4 tablespoons) coconut oil
60 chopped mallow leaves

Melt the oil, beeswax and coconut oil together over a low heat. Put in the mallow leaves and stir over a very gentle heat for 10 minutes. Strain the ointment into a pot, leave it to set and cool and cover it. This can also be used for veterinary purposes.

For coughs, bronchitis and asthma: Soak 15 g (½ oz) mallow leaves and flowers in 1 litre (1¾ pints) water for 10 minutes. Bring them to just under boiling point, take them from the heat and let them stand for 10 minutes. Strain and drink as required, sweetened with honey if wished.

For inflammation of the mouth and throat: Use the above infusion as a gargle.

To reduce inflammation elsewhere: Steep mallow leaves in hot water for 2 minutes and bind them onto the affected part.

For small mouth ulcers (aphthas): Put 20 ml (4 teaspoons) each chopped mallow and white dead-nettle flowers and leaves into a saucepan with 1 litre (1¾ pints) cold water. Bring them to the boil, boil for 5 minutes and strain. Wash the mouth out with the decoction, holding it in the mouth as long as possible. Spit it out. Drink a cupful of the unused decoction.

A gargle for throat infections: Put 25 g (1 oz) each mallows, sage, rue and elderflowers into a saucepan with 575 ml (1 pint) water. Bring them to the boil and boil for 15 minutes. Add 15 ml (1 tablespoon) each cider vinegar and honey and boil for a further 5 minutes. Strain and bottle. Use 60 ml (4 tablespoons) to gargle with and spit it out. Drink 15 ml (1 tablespoon) of the unused mixture.

For toothache and painful gums: Chew a few flowers and leaves that have previously been softened by steeping them in warm water for 5 minutes.

For bee and wasp stings: Crush a few mallow leaves with olive or sunflower oil and apply them to the sting.

GOOD KING HENRY

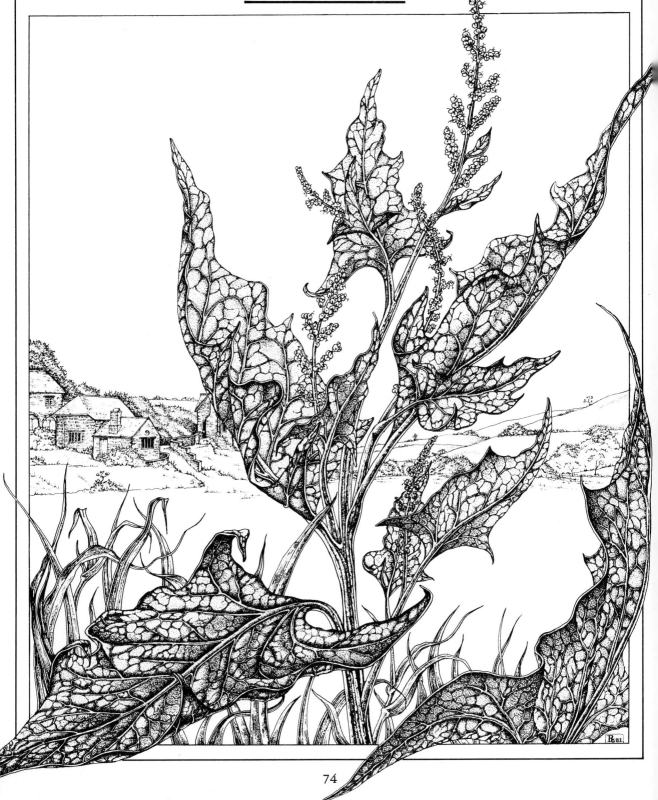

Availability

Good King Henry grows throughout the lowland regions of Britain, Scandinavia and Europe, being more common in the south. It grows throughout the United States, but not in mountainous areas. Though not found wild in Australasia, it can be easily cultivated and is available at herb nurseries.

Good King Henry thrives in rich pastures and arable land. It can also be found near the sites of old buildings, walls and gardens, since it was once cultivated as a pot-herb and garden vegetable.

It is very easily transplanted into the herb or vegetable garden but it is best if you let it become established for about 6 months before you start to pick it.

The leaves of Good King Henry can be picked all through early summer, until the plants start to get leggy (in May and June in the northern hemisphere/November and December in Australasia). Pick or cut off the whole leaves and wash them well when you get home. If you want to keep them for a few days before cooking them, pack them, quite wet, in a plastic bag and store them in the bottom of the refrigerator.

Stir-Fried Good King Henry

Stir-fry Good King Henry in the same way as fat hen (page 87), adding the same flavourings. It will cook down in exactly the same way.

Good King Henry with Spring Greens (Collards)

225g (8oz) Good King Henry
450g (1lb) spring greens (collards)
25g (1oz) butter
200ml (7fl oz) water

Wash and finely chop both vegetables. Melt the butter in a saucepan on a high heat. Turn the chopped leaves in the water to get them well coated. Pour in the water and bring it to the boil.

Cover the pan, lower the heat to moderate and cook the vegetables for 15 minutes, turning them once and adding a little more water if necessary. Drain them before serving. Serves 4.

Good King Henry and Sorrel Soup

Good King Henry and sorrel make a refreshing soup.

50g (2oz) Good King Henry leaves
16 large sorrel leaves
25g (1oz) butter
2 medium onions, finely chopped
15ml (1 tablespoon) wholewheat flour
850ml (1½ pints) stock
sea salt and freshly ground black pepper
100ml (3½fl oz) thick cream

Finely chop the Good King Henry and sorrel leaves. Melt the butter in a saucepan on a low heat.

Stir in the onions and cook them until they are golden. Stir in the flour and cook it for 1 minute. Stir in the stock, season and bring it to the boil. Stir in the sorrel and Good King Henry. Turn the heat to the lowest setting and cook the soup, uncovered, for 20 minutes. Stir in the cream just before serving. Serves 4.

Good King Henry with Bacon and Eggs

This is a variation on stir-fried Good King Henry. It makes a substantial main meal, but for a lunch or supper dish you can omit the eggs.

225g (8oz) Good King Henry
450g (1lb) green bacon
1 large onion
25g (1oz) butter
4 eggs

Wash and chop the Good King Henry. Finely chop the bacon. Quarter and thinly slice the onion.

Melt the butter in a frying pan on a moderate heat. Put in the bacon and onion and stir them around until the onion is soft. Put in the Good King Henry and keep stirring until it has cooked down and softened.

Put the bacon and Good King Henry into either a flat serving dish or onto four individual plates. Keep them warm.

Fry or poach the eggs and set them on top. Serves 4.

Buttered Good King Henry and Spinach

Good King Henry is excellent when mixed with other vegetables and this is very useful if you can only find a few plants.

350 g (12 oz) Good King Henry
350 g (12 oz) spinach
25 g (1 oz) butter

Wash and shake dry the leaves of both vegetables and break off the stems where they join the leaves.

Melt the butter in a saucepan on a moderate heat. Turn the leaves in the butter to get them well coated. Cover them and keep them on a low heat for 15 minutes, turning them once. If necessary, drain them in a collander before serving. Serves 4.

Medicinal

To cleanse and heal sores: Chop 225 g (8 oz) Good King Henry leaves and boil them in a very little water for 3 minutes. Drain them and lay them between two pieces of muslin. Lay them on the affected part.

Veterinary

Chickens will fatten quickly if fed the leaves of Good King Henry. The roots of the plant can be given to sheep for coughs.

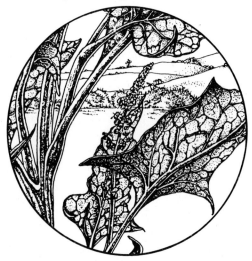

MARSH SAMPHIRE

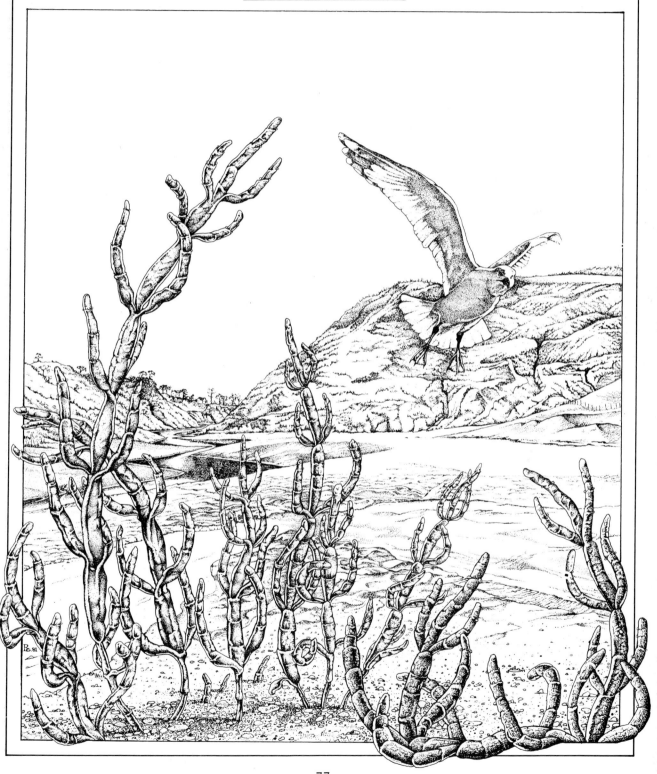

Availability

Marsh samphire grows all round the coasts of Britain, Europe and the United States, around estuaries and on salt marshes and mud flats. It tends to prefer spots where the mud is covered with a thin layer of shingle and the most succulent plants grow just below the tide line.

There is a saying that marsh samphire is ready for picking on the longest day of the year, but it is sometimes tall enough about a week before. For pickling and for making into sauces and serving as a side vegetable, pick the samphire young, when it is about four inches high and bright green and there is no "string" growing through the centre of the stem. For eating as a first course, wait until the plants are six to eight inches high and the string has just developed. In late summer (after the end of July in the northern hemisphere) the whole plants are generally too tough to pick, but for sauces and for pickling you can take off just the side shoots.

Marsh samphire is best gathered by cutting it with scissors. Hold the tops of several stems with one hand and cut them off at the base. Breaking off each piece separately takes a good deal of time and in gathering it that way you can easily pull out the small root.

Before cooking, wash the samphire well in cold water and drain it. Never soak it for this makes it decay quickly. It will keep, unwashed and quite dry, in a plastic bag in the bottom of the refrigerator for up to 3 days.

A First Course of Marsh Samphire

For this, pick marsh samphire when it is six to eight inches high and the thin "string" has developed through the centre of the stem.

Bring a large pan of unsalted water to the boil and, for four to six people, plunge in 450 g (1 lb) samphire. Boil it for 7 minutes and drain it.

Have ready to serve with it, melted butter, a vinaigrette dressing or Hollandaise sauce. The idea is to eat the samphire with your fingers, rather as you would a globe artichoke. Pick up a stem and dip it in the butter or sauce. Then scrape the fleshy part from the string with your teeth and tongue. Delicious.

Marsh Samphire in Cream

This rich, extravagant recipe is best with plainly cooked lamb or boiled bacon.

225 g (8 oz) young marsh samphire
150 ml (¼ pint) thick cream
60 ml (4 tablespoons) chopped parsley
freshly ground black pepper

Drop the samphire into boiling water and cook it for 1 minute. Drain it.

Put the cream into a saucepan and bring it to just below boiling point. Put in the samphire and parsley and season with a liberal amount of black pepper. Cover and simmer the samphire gently for 2 minutes. Serve it hot. Serves 4.

Marsh Samphire Salad

This salad is best with cold lamb or pork. Pick the samphire right at the beginning of its season and use the youngest, tenderest shoots.

25 g (1 oz) young marsh samphire shoots
30 ml (2 tablespoons) chopped chives
60 ml (4 tablespoons) olive oil
30 ml (2 tablespoons) cider vinegar
1.5 ml (¼ teaspoon) dried mustard powder
5 ml (1 teaspoon) honey
freshly ground black pepper
1 lettuce

Finely chop the samphire and put it into a salad bowl with the chives. Add the oil, vinegar, mustard, honey and pepper and stir well to make a thick dressing.

Wash and dry the lettuce and tear it into small pieces. Gently fold it into the dressing so every piece becomes well-coated and the samphire is evenly distributed. Serves 4.

Samphire Sauce for Roast Lamb

25 g (1 oz) young marsh samphire
150 ml (¼ pint) dry red wine
30 ml (2 tablespoons) red wine vinegar
60 ml (4 tablespoons) chopped mint

Finely chop the samphire. After you have roasted your joint of lamb, pour away any excess fat from the roasting tin. Set the tin on top of the stove on a moderate heat. Pour in the wine and bring it to the boil, scraping in any residue from the bottom of the tin. Stir in the vinegar, samphire and mint and simmer the sauce for 2 minutes.

Serve it separately as you would a plain mint sauce. Serves 4.

Marsh Samphire Mayonnaise

This mayonnaise goes best with shellfish and white fish.

25 g (1 oz) young marsh samphire
1 egg yolk
2.5 ml (½ teaspoon) dried mustard powder
freshly ground black pepper
125 ml (4 fl oz) olive oil
up to 30 ml (2 tablespoons) white wine vinegar
45 ml (3 tablespoons) chopped parsley

Drop the samphire into unsalted boiling water and boil it for 1 minute. Drain it in a collander, run cold water through it. Cool it completely and finely chop it.

Put the egg yolk into a bowl with the mustard powder and a few grindings of pepper. Drop by drop, beat in 30 ml (2 tablespoons) of the oil and then 10 ml (2 teaspoons) of the vinegar, 5 ml (1 teaspoon) at a time. Gradually add the rest of the oil and then more vinegar to taste. Fold in the chopped samphire and the parsley.

Sweet Pickle of Samphire

350 g (12 oz) young marsh samphire
425 ml (¾ pint) light cider vinegar
10 ml (2 teaspoons) mustard seeds
10 ml (2 teaspoons) black peppercorns
2 dried chillies
1 piece root ginger, bruised
125 g (4 oz) honey

Put the vinegar into an enamelled or stainless steel saucepan with the mustard seeds, peppercorns, chillies and root ginger. Let it stand for 1 hour. Bring it to the boil, boil it for 10 minutes and strain it.

Blanch the samphire by dropping it into boiling water and cooking it for one minute. Strain it and pack it into a 450 g (1 lb) jar.

Return the vinegar to its saucepan. Put in the honey and stir over a low heat for it to dissolve. Boil the syrup for 5 minutes and skim it if necessary. Pour it over the samphire and cover the jar immediately.

Keep the pickle for 1 week before opening. Fills one 450 g (1 lb) jar.

MEADOWSWEET

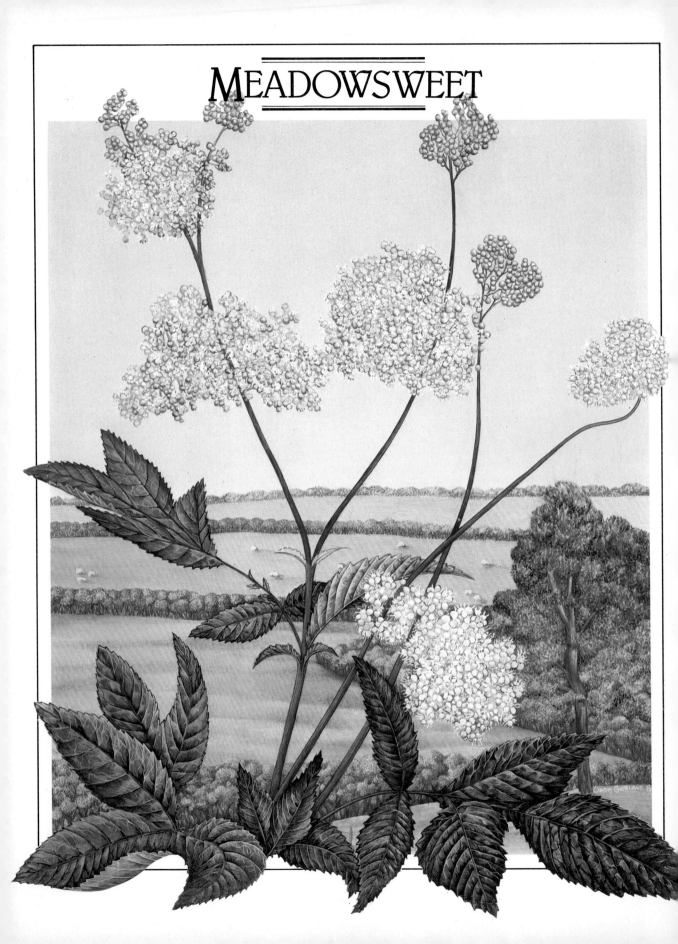

FILIPENDULA ULMARIA

Local Names: Bittersweet, Bridewort, Courtship and Matrimony, Dolloff, Hayriff, Kiss-me-Quick, Lady-of-the-Meadow, Maid-of-the-Meadow, Maid-of-the-Mead, May of the Meadow, Meadow Queen, Meadsweet, Mead-Soot, Meadwort, New Mown Hay, Queen of the Meadow, Queen's Feather, Summer's Farewell, Sweet Hay, Tea-Flower, Wireweed.

Availability

Meadowsweet grows throughout Britain, Scandinavia and Europe. In America it is grown as a cultivated plant in gardens, but it can also be found growing wild, mainly in the mid-western states. Also in America grows a related species, Regina prati or Queen of the Prairies, which can be used in the same ways. In Australasia, it is not found wild but can be easily grown.

Meadowsweet thrives best in damp places such as wet meadows, damp woods, fens, ditches, wet roadside verges, marshes and swamps.

Pick meadowsweet from early to late summer (late June and early July in the northern hemisphere/December and January in Australasia), when the softly sweet smelling flowers are fully open.

The stems are very brittle so, if you have forgotten your scissors, you can carefully break them, giving you whole sprays of leaves and flowers about 30–35 cm (15–18 inches) long.

Meadowsweet with Tart Fruits

If you put meadowsweet into the saucepan when you are cooking tart fruits, it not only gives them a delicious, honeyed flavour, but also gives the impression that they are sweetened with honey. Consequently, you need to add far less honey or sugar to sweeten the fruits.

You can serve the fruits plainly, with cream or custard or use them as a base for a more complicated dish such as a mousse or fruit fool.

Use meadowsweet to sweeten apples, apricots, black and red currants, gooseberries and plums. Use 4 flower heads to every 450g (1lb) fruit. Sweet white wine will also reduce the need for a sweetener.

Meadowsweet with Apricots

450g (1lb) apricots
125ml (4fl oz) sweet white wine
4 heads meadowsweet flowers

Stone the apricots and slice them lengthways. Put them into a saucepan with the wine and meadowsweet flowers.

Set them on a low heat and bring them to simmering point. Cover them and cook them gently for 15 minutes so they are tender but still firm.

Remove the flower heads and serve the apricots hot or cold. Serves 4.

Meadowsweet Ice Cream

Make as Woodruff ice cream (page 53) using one meadowsweet flower head.

Meadowsweet with Gooseberries

450g (1lb) gooseberries
125ml (4fl oz) sweet white wine or water
15ml (1 tablespoon) honey
4 heads meadowsweet flowers

Top and tail the gooseberries.
Put the wine and honey into a saucepan and set them on a low heat. Stir for the honey to melt. Put in the gooseberries and meadowsweet flowers.

Cover the pan and cook the gooseberries on a low heat for 15 minutes so they are soft but still whole.

Serve them hot or cold. Custard goes with them beautifully. Serves 4.

Meadowsweet Aperitif

Once you have drunk this before a meal, any other aperitif will fade into second place!

1 bottle claret
3 flower heads of meadowsweet
1 meadowsweet leaf, bruised

Pour the wine into a jug. Put in the flower heads and leaves and leave for 2 hours. Strain the wine into a decanter and serve it at room temperature.

Meadowsweet Tea

A tea made from the fresh or dried flowers is fragrant and soothing. One made with only the leaves is more refreshing. You can also mix flowers and leaves.

To make the tea, infuse 1 fresh flower head or four shredded fresh leaves in 225ml (8fl oz) boiling water for 10 minutes. If using dried meadowsweet, use 5ml (1 teaspoon) crumbled flowers or leaves or a mixture.

Meadowsweet Beer

This is a light, refreshing beer.

125 g (4 oz) meadowsweet leaves
450 g (1 lb) malt extract
225 g (8 oz) light brown (demerara) sugar
4.6 litres (1 gallon) water
15 g (½ oz) dried yeast
2.5 ml (½ teaspoon) brown sugar per 575 ml (1 pint)
  bottle

Boil the meadowsweet leaves in 1.725 litres (3 pints) water for 15 minutes. Dissolve the malt and sugar in a further 1.725 litres (3 pints) water in a large container. Strain the meadowsweet liquid onto the malt and sugar, reserving the meadowsweet.

Boil the meadowsweet for a further 10 minutes in 1.15 litres (2 pints) water. Strain the liquid onto the malt and sugar solution, this time discarding the meadowsweet.

Cool the liquid to lukewarm and sprinkle the yeast on top. Leave the beer, covered, until it begins to ferment. Then put it into a warm place for three days, or until fermentation stops.

Rack off the beer and bottle it, adding 2.5 ml (½ teaspoon) sugar to each 575 ml (1 pint) bottle. Seal tightly and leave the beer undisturbed until it is clear (about 1 week) before opening.

Medicinal

For headaches: Infuse 10 ml (2 teaspoons) dried mixed meadowsweet flowers and leaves in 225 ml (8 fl oz) just under boiling water for 15 minutes. Drink the whole amount twice a day.

To lower a temperature which accompanies a cold, a chill or influenza: Infuse 10 ml (2 teaspoons) dried flowers and leaves in 225 ml (8 fl oz) just under boiling water for 10 minutes. Strain and drink the whole amount twice a day.

To reduce fever: Boil 45 ml (3 tablespoons) meadowsweet flowers in 1 litre (1¾ pints) dry white wine for 10 minutes. Strain. Allow the wine to settle, covered, for 24 hours and then bottle it. Drink a small aperitif glass of the wine every 2 hours.

For rheumatism: Infuse 75 ml (5 tablespoons) dried mixed flowers and leaves in 1 litre (1¾ pints) just under boiling water for 10 minutes. Strain. Drink a cupful before meals and also apply the same infusion as a compress on the aching limb.

For diarrhoea in children: Infuse 25 g (1 oz) dried leaves in 575 ml (1 pint) just under boiling water for 10 minutes. Strain and sweeten with honey and give in wineglassful doses.

To dry up sores and ulcers: Boil 40 g (1½ oz) leaves in ½ litre (16 fl oz) water for 10 minutes. Take them off the heat and let them stand for 10 minutes. Strain and bathe the affected part.

Veterinary

Meadowsweet is a favourite bee plant.
For fevers and diarrhoea in animals, infuse 2 handfuls chopped flowers in 1.15 litres (2 pints) water for 15 minutes. Strain and add 30 ml (2 tablespoons) honey. Give it to the animal to drink throughout the day, without food.

WILD STRAWBERRY

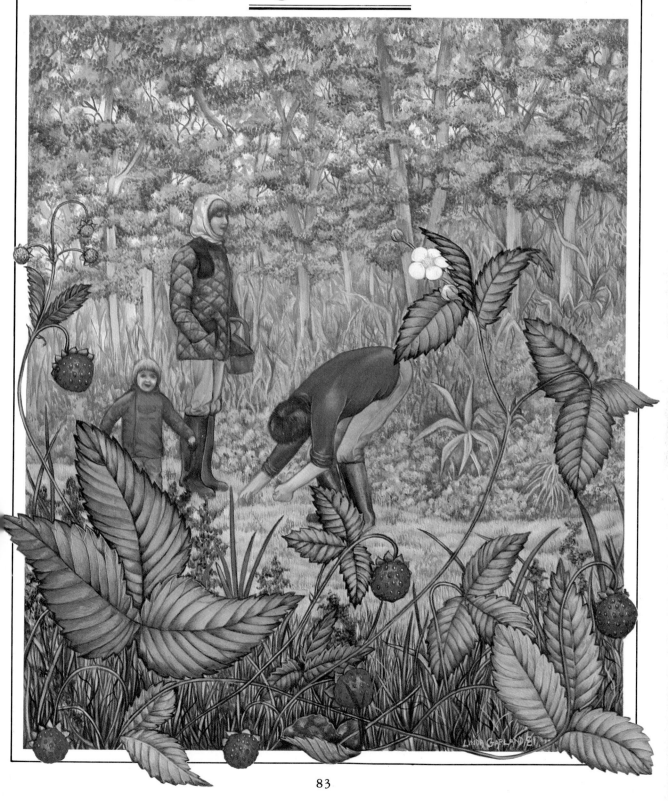

Availability

The wild strawberry grows throughout Britain, Scandinavia, Europe and Australasia. In America, it grows mainly in the mid-western and southern states.

The best places to find wild strawberries are grassy banks and heaths, in open woodland and by country lanes. They flourish best where the grass and other plants around them are fairly low.

The tiny fruits can be picked all through summer, but it is rare that you will be able to pick great quantities since only a few on each plant ripen at one time. Pick them like cultivated strawberries, without hulling them.

Leaves of wild strawberries can also be picked throughout the summer months. Take only one or two from each plant.

The roots for medicinal purposes, should be lifted in early spring (March in the northern hemisphere/September in Australasia).

Strawberry Leaf Tea

This tastes sweet and delicate and should be made with the dried leaves. Infuse 15 ml (1 tablespoon) crushed dried strawberry leaves in 575 ml (1 pint) boiling water for 10 minutes. Strain the liquid and sweeten it, if required, with honey.

Melon and Strawberries

2 cantaloup melons
225 g (8 oz) very ripe cultivated strawberries
up to 225 g (8 oz) wild strawberries

Cut the melons in half crossways and scoop out the seeds. Put each melon half into a separate dish.

Rub the cultivated strawberries through a sieve. Spoon the resulting purée into the hollows of the melon halves and also in a thin stream round the cut edges.

Scatter the wild strawberries in the centre and round the edges.

Serve as a first course or as a dessert.

Wild Strawberry Syllabub

If you can't find enough wild strawberries for this deliciously simple sweet, make up the amount with fresh raspberries.

Hawthorn essence (page 67) can be used instead of
  brandy or whisky.
275 ml (½ pint) thick cream
30 ml (2 tablespoons) brandy or whisky
15 ml (1 tablespoon) honey
250 g (8 oz) wild strawberries

Whip the cream until it stands in soft peaks and whip in the spirit and honey. Fold in the strawberries and divide the syllabub between four chilled glasses. Serves 4.

Wild Strawberries, Peaches and Cream

6 medium sized peaches
150 ml (¼ pint) thick cream
30 ml (2 tablespoons) honey
125 g (4 oz) wild strawberries, or as many as you have

Scald and skin the peaches. Stone and thinly slice four of them and divide them between four glass dishes. Stone the remaining two peaches and either rub them through a sieve or work them in a blender to a smooth purée.

Stiffly whip the cream and whip in the peach purée and honey. Spoon the peach cream over the peach slices.

Scatter the wild strawberries over the top. Serves 4.

Wild Strawberry and Walnut Shortcakes

40 g (1½ oz) walnuts
150 g (5 oz) flour
40 g (1½ oz) light brown (demerara) sugar
2 drops vanilla extract
125 g (4 oz) butter, softened
275 ml (½ pint) thick cream
125 g (4 oz) wild strawberries, or as many as you have

Heat the oven to Reg 4/180C/350F.
Finely chop the walnuts and put them into a bowl with the flour, sugar and vanilla extract. Cut in the butter and, with your fingers, work the mixture to a smooth dough.

Roll the dough out to 6 mm (¼ inch) thick and cut it into 5 cm (2 inch) rounds with a biscuit cutter. Lay them on a floured baking sheet and bake them for 25 minutes, so they just begin to brown. Lift them onto wire racks to cool.

Stiffly whip the cream. You will have 20–24 biscuits (cookies) so use only enough for the amount of wild strawberries that you have. The rest will keep well in an airtight tin for another day. Pile the whipped cream on top of the biscuits and decorate them with wild strawberries.

Wild Strawberry Flan

If you haven't enough wild strawberries to fill the flan case, make a ring round the edge of the hollow first with slices of fresh apricots.

125 g (4 oz) butter, softened
125 g (4 oz) honey
125 g (4 oz) wholewheat flour
2.5 ml (½ teaspoon) baking powder
2 eggs, beaten
butter for greasing an 18 cm (7 inch) flan case that has the central part of the base raised
60 ml (4 tablespoons) redcurrant jelly
15 ml (1 tablespoon) dry red wine
175 g (6 oz) wild strawberries
whipped cream for serving (optional)

Heat the oven to Reg 6/200C/400F. Beat the butter to a cream and then beat in the honey. Toss the flour with the baking powder and beat it into the butter and honey, alternately with the eggs. Put the mixture into the buttered flan case tin and bake it for 20 minutes, or until the sponge is browned and has shrunk slightly from the sides of the tin. Turn it onto a wire rack to cool.

Beat the redcurrant jelly with a fork so it is almost liquid. Put it into a saucepan with the wine and melt it. Brush the hollow of the flan with redcurrant jelly and keep the remaining melted jelly warm. Put the strawberries into the flan and brush them thickly with the remaining glaze. If any glaze is left, brush the sides and edges of the flan so the whole has a shiny red appearance. Serve plainly or with whipped cream. Serves 6.

Wild Strawberry and Cream Cheese Tartlets

This is another adaptable recipe, enabling you to use even a very small amount of wild strawberries.

shortcrust pastry made with 125 g (4 oz) wholewheat flour
175 g (6 oz) sweet cream cheese
30 ml (2 tablespoons) soured cream
15 ml (1 tablespoon) honey
as many wild strawberries as you can gather

Heat the oven to Reg 6/200C/400F. Make the pastry and use it to line 12 small tartlet tins. Bake the pastry shells for 15 minutes, turn them out and cool them.

Put the cream cheese into a bowl and beat in the soured cream and the honey. Spoon the mixture into the tartlet cases.

Decorate the heaps of cream cheese filling with wild strawberries. If you have only 12, put one on top of each. If more, make patterns on the tarts with them. If you have enough, you can even make a pyramid of strawberries on each tart.

Medicinal

To cool a sunburnt face: Rub it with a cut wild strawberry. Or, rub some wild strawberries through a sieve and use them as a face pack, leaving them on for 30 minutes. Wash it off with warm water to which you have added a few drops of simple tincture of benzoin.

For inflamed patches on the skin, skin rashes and inflamed eyes: Chop wild strawberry leaves and soak them in hot water for 2 minutes. Put them between two pieces of muslin and apply them as a poultice.

To prevent chilblains: Rub the parts likely to be affected during the winter with crushed wild strawberries and if possible use the strawberries as a poultice, leaving them on overnight.

For anaemia: Wild strawberries have a high assimilable iron content, so eat them as often as possible.

For heavy or prolonged menstruation: Infuse 45 ml (3 tablespoons) chopped wild strawberry leaves in 1 litre (1¼ pints) boiling water for 5 minutes. Strain, and drink a cupful, sweetened with honey if required, three times a day.

For diarrhoea and dysentery: Make a decoction by boiling 45 ml (3 tablespoons) chopped strawberry roots in 1 litre (1¾ pints) water for 10 minutes. Strain. Drink 1 cupful first thing in the morning and another last thing at night.

FAT HEN

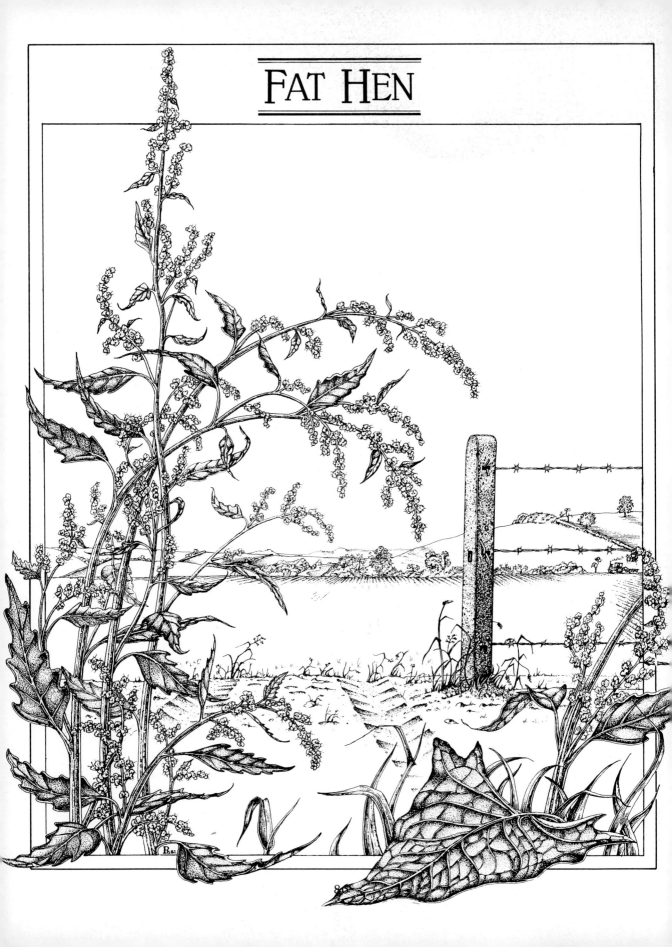

CHENOPODIUM ALBUM

Local Names: All Good, Bacon Weed, Confetti,
Dirty Dick/Jack/John, Dung Weed, Frost-Blite, Lamb's
Quarters, Melsweed, Midden Myles, Muckweed, Mutton
Chops, Mutton Tops, Pigweed, Rag Jack, White Goosefoot,
Wild Pottage.

Availability

Fat hen grows throughout Britain, Scandinavia, Europe, Australasia and the United States in all but mountainous areas.

It grows easily on disturbed ground such as sites of house building and road works besides garden and cultivated agricultural land. It flourishes best on very rich soil such as that around manure heaps and farm yards and well-composted garden plots.

In very early summer, the whole of the plant can be picked and used. After this, pick only the leaves and tops since the stalks will have become too tough. When the green flowers appear later (late June in the northern hemisphere/December in Australasia) these may be cooked with the rest of the plant. If you have enough of them they can be cooked like broccoli, but just a few will disappear into the leaves when cooked. You can continue picking the leaves in all for about a month (until the beginning of July in the northern hemisphere/ January in Australasia). After this the plants become too straggly and the leaves sparse.

Wash fat hen well before cooking. If you are not able to use it all at once, store it, quite wet, in a polythene bag in the bottom of the refrigerator. It will stay fresh for about five days.

When cooking fat hen, remember that the enormous amount that you first put into the pan will very soon cook down to about a quarter of its original bulk.

Fat Hen in Salads

A few chopped, young fat hen leaves added to a green salad give a fresh, nutty flavour.

Fat Hen as a Vegetable

There are three basic ways of cooking fat hen as a vegetable: boiling, buttering and stir-frying.

Boiled fat hen is rather like boiled spinach with a mild flavour and moist texture. Buttering gives a similar texture but slightly stronger flavour.

450 g (1 lb) fat hen will only feed two people as a single vegetable. If you are boiling or buttering and have a really large saucepan, you can increase the amounts, but it is impossible to stir-fry more than 450 g (1 lb) at a time because of the original bulk. It is best to just have a little each and accompany it with another vegetable.

Stir-Fried Fat Hen

Wash 450 g (1 lb) fat hen and chop it finely. In a really large frying pan or paella pan, melt 25 g (1 oz) butter on a high heat. Mix in the fat hen and keep stirring it around on the heat until it cooks down and becomes soft, bright green and glossy. This will take 3–4 minutes. Serve it as soon as you can.

An onion can be stir-fried for about 1 minute in the butter before you add the fat hen. A little chopped rosemary or thyme or some chopped chives or spring onions can be added with the leaves. Nutmeg can be grated on during cooking.

Fat Hen and Cheese Tart

Well-flavoured, stir-fried fat hen, like spinach, makes a good filling for a tart.

shortcrust pastry made with 225 g (8 oz) wholewheat flour
450 g (1 lb) fat hen
25 g (1 oz) butter
2 medium onions, thinly sliced
1 clove garlic, finely chopped
sea salt and freshly ground black pepper
45 ml (3 tablespoons) chopped parsley
45 ml (3 tablespoons) chopped thyme
5 ml (1 teaspoon) chopped rosemary
¼ nutmeg, grated
125 g (4 oz) Cheddar cheese, grated
6 eggs, beaten

Make the pastry and chill it slightly. Finely chop the fat hen. Melt the butter in a very large frying pan or paella pan on a high heat. Mix in the onions and stir them around until they are beginning to brown. Mix in the garlic and then the fat hen. Keep stirring the fat hen until it is soft and glossy and has cooked down. Take the pan from the heat and mix in the seasonings, herbs and nutmeg. Leave the fat hen to cool.

Roll out the pastry and use it to line a 25 cm (10 inch) diameter flan tin. Put in the fat hen in an even layer and scatter the cheese over the top. Pour in the eggs, making sure they are evenly distributed. Bake the tart for 30 minutes so the top is golden. Serve it hot. Serves 4–6.

Boiled Fat Hen

Wash the fat hen and leave the leaves and smaller sprigs whole. Bring 5 cm (2 inches) water to the boil in a saucepan. Put in the fat hen and press it down well. Cover and simmer for 10 minutes. Drain the fat hen, pressing down well to extract as much water as possible.

Buttered Fat Hen

Again, leave the leaves and smaller sprigs whole. To each 450 g (1 lb) fat hen, melt 25 g (1 oz) butter in a saucepan on a high heat. Put in the fat hen, a little at a time, and turn it in the butter. When it is well coated, turn the heat to the lowest temperature, cover the pan and cook the fat hen for 10 minutes, stirring once. Drain it, if necessary, before serving.

A chopped onion or several chopped spring onions (scallions) can be softened in the butter before putting in the fat hen and various herbs such as thyme or a very little rosemary can be added with the leaves.

Sautéed Fat Hen with Nutmeg

This dries out boiled fat hen and gives it a richer texture.

450 g (1 lb) fat hen
25 g (1 oz) butter
¼ nutmeg, grated

Boil the fat hen as above and drain it well. Melt the butter in a frying pan on a high heat. Put in the fat hen and chop it into the butter. Keep stirring and chopping until it is quite dry and glossy. Grate in the nutmeg and serve as soon as possible.

Fat Hen Soup with Soured Cream and Pine Kernels

This is a smooth, deep green soup. The pine kernels not only look attractive but also make a good contrast in flavour and texture. You can, however, omit them for family meals and use parsley instead.

450 g (1 lb) fat hen
1 large onion
575 ml (1 pint) stock
sea salt and freshly ground black pepper
¼ nutmeg, grated
1 clove garlic, crushed with a pinch sea salt
25 g (1 oz) butter
30 ml (2 tablespoons) wholewheat flour
150 ml (¼ pint) milk
150 ml (¼ pint) soured cream
25 g (1 oz) pine nuts, toasted until brown

Chop the fat hen and the onion. Bring the stock to the boil in a large saucepan. Put in the fat hen and the onion and season with the salt, pepper and nutmeg. Cover and simmer for 10 minutes.

Take the pan from the heat and cool the contents a little. Then work them in a blender so you have a smooth, deep green purée. Put in the garlic and blend again.

Melt the butter in the cleaned saucepan on a moderate heat. Stir in the flour and cook it for ½ minute. Stir in the milk and stir until you have a thick, bubbling sauce. Stir in the fat hen purée and bring the soup to simmering point. Stir in the soured cream.

Pour the soup into individual bowls and float the pine kernels in the centre. Serves 4.

Medicinal

Eat fat hen in the early summer as a general tonic. It contains more iron and protein than cabbage or spinach.

Veterinary

The leaves, flowers and seeds of fat hen make a valuable poultry food. When the seed heads are ripe they make a good food for caged birds and will keep them free from worms.

WILD ROSE

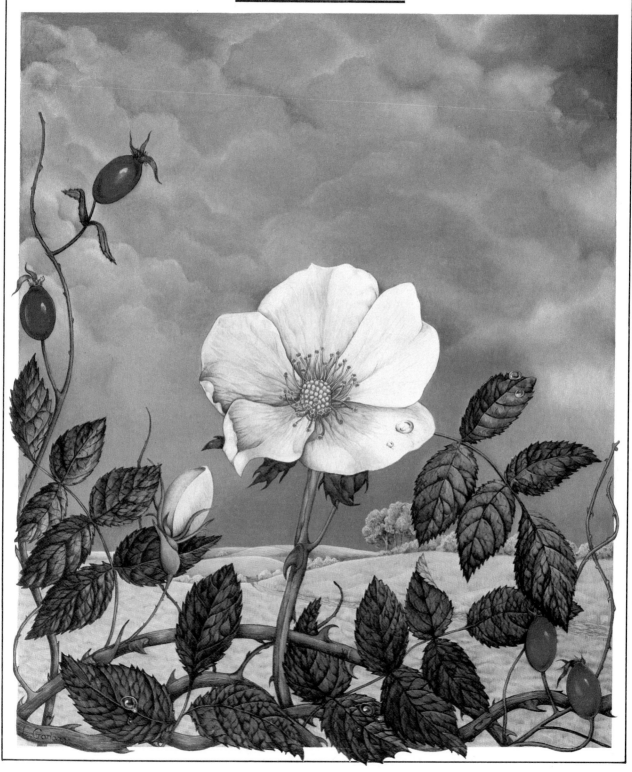

Availability

The wild rose grows throughout Great Britain, although to a lesser extent in Scotland; in Europe, the United States, Canada, Australia and New Zealand. Both the petals and the bright orange-red fruits known as the hips can be used. The wild rose blooms all through summer (June to August in the northern hemisphere). Never pick the petals from a young flower but wait until they are just about to drop off naturally. To test for this, gently shake the full blown flower and see if any petals drop off.

Rose Hip Tart

450g (1 lb) rose hips
225g (8 oz) sugar
5 ml (1 teaspoon) ground cinnamon
5 ml (1 teaspoon) ground ginger
shortcrust pastry made with 175g (6 oz) wholemeal
 flour
beaten egg for glaze

Wash the hips, cut each one in half and scoop out and discard the seeds. Mix the outer husk with the sugar, cinnamon and ginger. Line an 18cm (7 inch) diameter flan tin with about two thirds of the pastry and fill it with the hips. Cover the plate with the remaining pastry, brush with beaten egg and bake it in a preheated oven Reg 6/200C/400F, for 30 minutes. Scatter the icing sugar over the top and serve it hot.

Rose Petal Sandwiches

15g (½ oz) fresh wild rose petals
125g (4 oz) unsalted butter

Lightly crush the petals and put half of them into a flat dish. Soften the butter and put it over the petals. Scatter the remaining petals over the top. Cover and leave overnight in a cool place. Scrape away the petals from the butter. Spread the butter over very thin slices of wholewheat bread which have the crusts removed. Cut the sandwiches into triangles. This makes a dainty tea time treat. A little honey may be spread over the butter if desired.

Rose Petal Jelly

10 large cooking apples
575 ml (1 pint) cold water
one 10cm (3 inch) piece cinnamon stick
thinly pared rind ½ lemon
225g (8 oz) sugar to every 275 ml (½ pint) liquid
25g (1 oz) fresh rose petals

Peel, core and slice the apples. Put them into a large saucepan with the water, cinnamon stick and lemon rind. Bring them to the boil and simmer them for 1½ hours until they are soft and pulpy. Strain the contents of the pan through a jelly bag and measure the liquid. Return it to the rinsed out pan. Gently warm the equivalent amount of sugar in a low oven. Stir it into the liquid and set the pan on a low heat until the sugar has dissolved. Bring to the boil, stir in the rose petals and stir until setting point is reached. Pour the jelly into hot, sterilised jars and cover it with rings of waxed paper. Cover it completely when it is set and cool. Use as a conserve with bread and buns or use it to fill sponge cakes.

Wine and Cordials

Rose Petal Tea

15 ml (1 tablespoon) dried wild rose petals
575 ml (1 pint) boiling water

Put the rose petals into a small pot and pour on the boiling water. Cover and infuse for 5 minutes. Strain and drink plain or sweetened with a little honey.

Rose Hip and Honey Syrup

This syrup is rich in Vitamin C and a little every day, diluted with hot water, will help to keep colds away. It is also delicious drunk purely for pleasure and undiluted it can be mixed with yoghurt or used as a sauce for puddings and ice creams.

2.5 kg (4 lbs) rose hips
5.5 litres (9 pints) water
honey: 450 g (1 lb) for every 850 ml (1½ pints) liquid

Bring two thirds of the water to the boil in a preserving pan. Mince the rose hips or finely chop them in a blender. Put them immediately into the boiling water. Bring them back to the boil, draw the pan aside and leave it for 15 minutes. Strain the liquid through a jelly bag. Put the pulp back into the pan, bring the rest of the water to the boil and pour it over the pulp. Stir and leave for 10 minutes. Strain the liquid and put it with the first batch. Measure the total amount and return it to the rinsed out pan with the corresponding amount of honey. Bring the syrup to the boil and boil for 5 minutes. Pour the syrup into hot, sterilised, dark bottles and cork immediately. The syrup can be used immediately but will keep for up to a year in a cool, dark place.

Rose Hip and Raisin Wine

for 4.6 litres (1 gallon):

1.8 kg (4 lbs) rose hips
900 g (2 lbs) raisins
1 lemon
1.35 kg (3 lbs) sugar
4.6 litres (1 gallon) water
yeast
yeast nutrient
pectolase

Mince the rose hips and raisins together. Put them into a plastic container with the juice and thinly pared rind of the lemon and the sugar. Bring the water to the boil and pour it over the hips and raisins. Stir. When the mixture is lukewarm add the yeast, yeast nutrient and pectolase. Cover and keep warm for a week. Strain the wine into a 4.6 litre (1 gallon) jar and fit a fermentation lock. Rack until the wine is clear, bottle it and leave it for a year before opening. The wine will be a rich, tawny brown and similar in flavour to a medium sherry.

Rose Hip Tea

Lay the hips out in a warm, airy room to dry. Then crush them into very small pieces. If you use metal to crush them make sure it is stainless steel. Otherwise use a large, wooden pestle and mortar. Store the crushed hips in an air- and light-tight jar. To make the tea, pour 575 ml (1 pint) boiling water over 10 ml (2 teaspoons) of the crushed hips. Infuse for 5–10 minutes and it will be a beautiful, deep pink colour.

Medicinal

Rose petal vinegar

For headaches after exposure to the sun.

one 369 ml (13 fl oz) bottle white wine vinegar
15 g (½ oz) dried or 25 g (1 oz) fresh wild rose petals

Pour out a little vinegar from the bottle to accomodate the petals. Push the petals into the jar, cover the jar and leave it on a sunny windowsill for three weeks.

To use the vinegar, dab it on the forehead and temples and lie down and relax for a while.

To remove liver spots from the skin: Crush dried rose hips (see tea) to a paste with water. Spread the paste over the liver spots. Leave it until it is dry and rinse it off with rose water.

For a soft complexion

15 ml (1 tablespoon) dried wild rose petals
30 ml (2 tablespoons) medium oatmeal

Fill a small muslin bag with the rose petals and oatmeal. When you run your bath, swish the bag about in the water. The bag may be used twice.

CARRAGHEEN MOSS

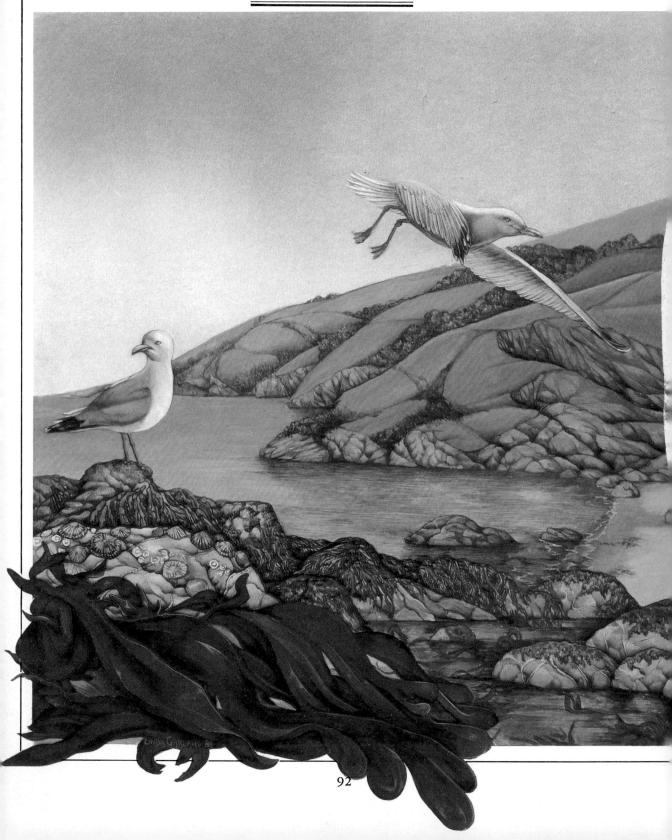

DULSE, LAVER

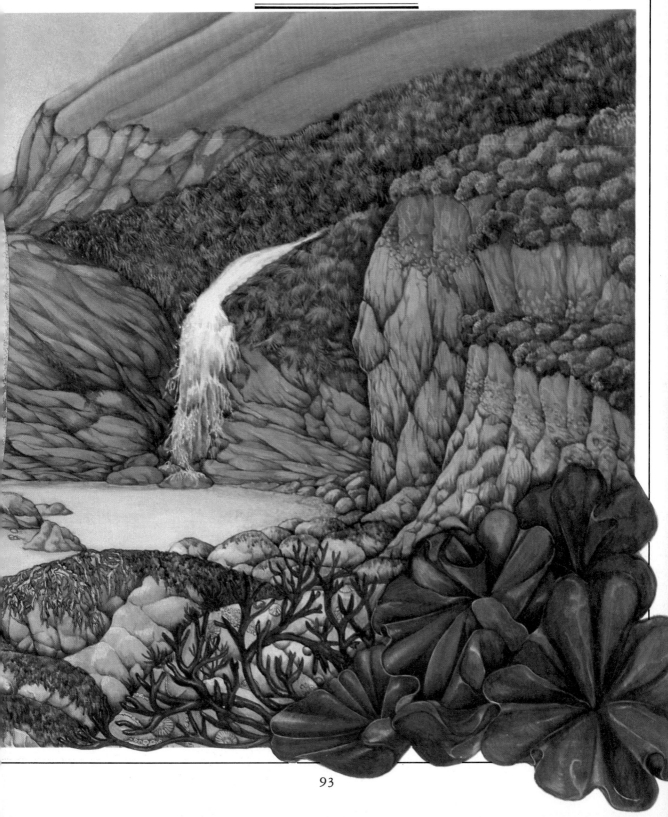

CARRAGHEEN

CHONDRUS CRISPUS

Local Names: Dorset Moss, Dorset Weed, Iberian Moss, Irish Moss, Salt Rock Moss

Availability

Carragheen can be found on the temperate Atlantic coasts of Britain, Europe and North America. It can also be found around the Channel Islands and occasionally on the English Channel and North Sea coasts of Britain and Europe. It is not common in Australasia but can be bought dried.

Carragheen grows on rocks and in rock pools that are below the tide line and it should be gathered in spring and early summer when it is young and soft. Cut the purple brown fan shapes of weed from the flat stems with scissors, leaving the stalk still attached to the rock to grow again. Always pick large amounts since carragheen shrinks enormously when it is dried. Take it home in a plastic bag and start processing it straight away.

To prepare carragheen for storing

It is more convenient to use carragheen if it has been dried, but first it is necessary to wash away the salt and to bleach it.

Lay an old sheet, several old cotton cloths sewn together or a large piece of muslin on a sheltered part of the lawn. Spread the carragheen on it in a single layer and anchor it down with garden netting. Leave it until it has bleached to a creamy white colour with a few pink edges (about 2 weeks). The salt needs to be washed out during bleaching so every day, if it does not rain, hose the carragheen down with water. After the final hosing, shake it dry and spread it out on wire racks covered with cotton or muslin cloths. Leave it on a sunny windowsill or put it into an airing cupboard until it is dry.

Cut off any tough pieces of stalk and store the carragheen in a dry place in paper bags or glass jars. It will last for a year.

Chocolate Blancmange

This sets well to a firm texture. It is very good with fresh fruits, particularly orange segments. You can, if wished, make a frothier textured blancmange by adding the egg as in the recipe below.

15 g (½ oz) dried carragheen
575 ml (1 pint) milk
5 cm (2 inch) piece cinnamon stick
1 chip nutmeg
2 pieces thinly pared orange rind
30 ml (2 tablespoons) drinking chocolate

Soak the carragheen in cold water for 15 minutes. Drain it and put it into a saucepan with the milk, cinnamon, nutmeg and orange rind. Bring them to the boil and simmer them for 30 minutes.

Strain well, pressing down hard on the carragheen and rubbing it slightly so the softer pieces are puréed and go through the sieve. Quickly mix in the drinking chocolate and stir so it is well incorporated. Pour the mixture into a dish and leave it in a cool place for 1 hour to set.

For everyday occasions, you can serve the blancmange plainly, from the dish. For special occasions, pour it into small pots or dishes to set and top each one with either a hazelnut or some chopped walnuts together with whipped cream. Serves 6.

Honey Blancmange

This recipe demonstrates an alternative method for jellying the milk to make blancmange. This, and the water-soaking method both achieve a good set, so use whichever way is the most convenient.

Adding the egg to the mixture makes a frothier, lighter textured blancmange.

15 g (½ oz) dried carragheen
575 ml (1 pint) milk
5 cm (2 inch) piece cinnamon stick
1 chip nutmeg
2 thinly pared strips lemon rind
2 thinly pared strips orange rind
30 ml (2 tablespoons) honey
little freshly grated nutmeg
1 egg
natural yoghurt and fresh soft fruits for serving

In a saucepan, soak the carragheen in the milk for 1 hour. Put in the cinnamon, nutmeg chip and orange and lemon rinds. Bring the milk slowly to the boil and simmer it, stirring frequently, for 30 minutes.

Strain the liquid, pressing down hard on the carragheen and rubbing it slightly so the softer pieces go through the sieve as a purée. Quickly stir in the honey and grated nutmeg.

Have the egg beaten until it is very light and frothy. Pour the hot mixture onto it, beating all the time (an electric beater is best) so the mixture becomes thick and frothed. Pour it into a serving bowl or into individual pots.

Leave the blancmange in a cool place for 1 hour to set. Serve it topped with natural yoghurt and chopped soft fruits such as peaches, apricots or strawberries. Serves 6.

Orange Desserts

Carragheen does not absolutely set fruit juice but turns it to a soft, thick purée that wraps itself deliciously round fresh fruit. Serve these plainly or with whipped cream.

15 g (½ oz) carragheen
575 ml (1 pint) orange juice
1 blade mace
3 medium sized oranges

Soak the carragheen in water for 30 minutes. Drain it and put it into a saucepan with the orange juice and mace. Bring it slowly to the boil and simmer gently for 45 minutes or until the orange juice thickens. Strain the juice, pressing down well on the carragheen, and cool it.

Cut the rind and pith from the oranges and chop the flesh. Divide it between 6 small glass dishes. Pour the cooled juice over the pieces of orange and put the dishes into the refrigerator for 2 hours for the juice to thicken. Serves 6.

Savoury Vegetable Jellies

These soft-textured savoury jellies make a light first course.

15 g (½ oz) dried carragheen
575 ml (1 pint) stock
30 ml (2 tablespoons) tomato purée
2 thinly pared strips lemon rind
1 bayleaf
salt and freshly ground black pepper
2 medium sized carrots
2 celery sticks
3 tomatoes
60 ml (4 tablespoons) chopped parsley
mayonnaise for serving

Soak the carragheen in the stock for 30 minutes. Put them into a saucepan with the tomato purée, lemon rind and bayleaf and season them well. Bring them slowly to the boil and simmer for 1 hour, stirring occasionally. Strain the liquid, pressing down hard and leave it to cool but not set.

Finely dice the carrots and celery and steam them for 20 minutes. Scald, skin, deseed and finely chop the tomatoes. Mix the vegetables with the parsley and divide them between 4 individual soufflé dishes. Pour the cooled liquid over the vegetables and put the dishes into the refrigerator for 2 hours for the jelly to set.

Serve the jellies topped with mayonnaise. Serves 4.

Medicinal

To soothe minor burns and scalds: Infuse 15 g (½ oz) dried carragheen and 5 ml (1 teaspoon) pekoe tea in 575 ml (1 pint) boiling water until the water is cold. Strain the liquid and apply it to the affected part.

A Soothing Hand Gel

1 large cucumber
25 g (1 oz) dried carragheen

Finely chop the cucumber and work it in a blender to a pulp. Tie the pulp in muslin and squeeze out the juice. Steep the carragheen in the juice for 1 hour. Bring them slowly to the boil and simmer them very gently for 30 minutes. Strain through a sieve, rubbing and pressing down hard to purée the softer pieces of carragheen.

Cool the gel, pot it and keep it refrigerated. It will keep fresh for up to a week. It is good for your hands after gardening and your body after sunbathing, making the skin remarkably smooth and silky.

A night time drink for insomnia or acid indigestion: Steep 15 g (½ oz) dried carragheen in cold water for 15 minutes. Put it into a saucepan with 1.15 litres (2 pints) milk and a thinly pared strip of lemon rind. Bring it slowly to the boil. Strain the drink into four mugs, without pressing down. Sweeten it with honey and drink on going to bed.

For coughs, colds and pulmonary complaints: Drink the above milk drink three times a day.

For kidney and bladder infections: Steep 15 g (½ oz) dried carragheen in cold water for 15 minutes. Drain it and boil it in 1.725 litres (3 pints) milk, or a mixture of milk and water, or just water, for 45 minutes, adding a cinnamon stick and a thinly pared strip of lemon rind for flavour if wished. Strain, without pressing down. Sweeten with honey to taste and drink as required.

Invalid Food

A jelly made with carragheen is rich in minerals and therefore better invalid food than an ordinary jelly.

Veterinary

In parts of Ireland, when fodder began to run out in spring, carragheen was given to calves as a food supplement.

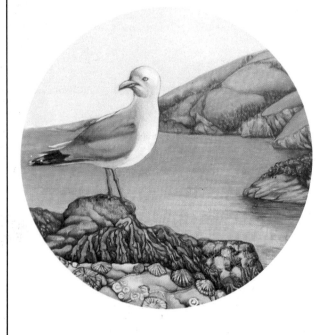

Availability

Dulse grows all round the Atlantic, North Sea and English Channel coasts of Britain, Europe and Scandinavia, and the Atlantic and Pacific coasts of America and Australasia.

The best time to collect dulse is in the early part of summer when it is still young. It can be gathered from below the tide line where you will find the red-brown, fan-like fronds attached to rocks and also, occasionally, to the stems of kelp. Cut off the fronds with sharp scissors, leaving the stem attached to the rock to grow again. If you are collecting dulse for drying, bear in mind that it will shrink considerably during the drying process.

To Dry Dulse

Wash it well to remove grit and small shells. Lay an old sheet, several cotton cloths sewn together or a large piece of muslin out on the lawn. Spread the dulse on it and anchor it down with garden netting. Leave it until it is dry and crisp. In case of very wet weather, start off the process outside and finish off the drying on a sunny windowsill or in the airing cupboard.

When the dulse is quite dry and crisp, store it in a dry place in paper bags or glass jars.

Stir-Fried Dulse

40 g (1½ oz) dried dulse
1 large onion
60 ml (4 tablespoons) sunflower oil
45 ml (3 tablespoons) tamari or soy sauce

Soak the dulse in cold water for 10 minutes. Drain it well. Thinly slice the onion. Heat the oil in a large frying pan or wok on a high heat. Put in the onion and stir it around until it begins to wilt. Put in the dulse and stir it for 2 minutes so it darkens in colour and softens. Mix in the sauce, let it bubble and take the pan from the heat. Serves 4.

Serving Stir-Fried Dulse

Stir-fried dulse can be eaten as a vegetable and it goes particularly well with lamb and white fish.

It can also be served with rice as a light supper or lunch dish and can be rolled into wholewheat pancakes.

Surprisingly, if left to go cold, it makes good sandwiches, used quite sparingly between slices of wholewheat bread.

Salt Substitute

Small pieces of dried dulse can be added to soups and stews to replace the salt.

Fried Rice and Dulse

This goes very well with eggs and fish dishes.

225 g (8 oz) brown rice
half quantity stir-fried dulse, as above
60 ml (4 tablespoons) sunflower oil
1 egg, beaten

Boil the rice in lightly salted water for 45 minutes, or until it is soft. Drain it, refresh it with cold water and drain it again. Finely chop the cooked dulse and mix it into the rice.

Heat the oil in a large frying pan or wok on a high heat. Mix in the rice and stir it about to heat it through. Mix in the egg and keep stirring until each rice grain acquires a fluffy coating. Serve as soon as possible. Serves 4.

Dulse Relish

Dulse has such a distinctive flavour that it really needs no other ingredients to boost or complement it. Serve this relish with plainly cooked oily fish such as grilled/broiled mackerel, or fried, oatmeal-coated herrings. You will only need a very little with each mouthful to give you a flavour of the sea.

15 g (½ oz) dried dulse
90 ml (6 tablespoons) white wine vinegar

Soak the dulse in the vinegar for 30 minutes. Drain it well and chop it finely. Serve it in a small dish.

Dulse Appetizer

Tear dried dulse into small pieces and serve it with drinks before a meal as you would salted nuts. It tastes extremely pleasant and goes very well with dry Martini.

LAVER

PORPHYRA UMBILICALIS
Local Names: Purple Laver, Sea Spinach, Sloke. (In Japan it is called Nori and the dried version may be sold as such in healthfood shops.)

Availability

Laver grows on the North Atlantic and North Sea coasts of Britain and Europe and also round the Mediterranean Sea. There are two related species of Porphyra in the United States and Australasia which can be used in the same ways.

Laver grows on rocks and stones, usually between middle and low tide levels. It does not have a particular season but will come and go at intervals, so it is best to always keep a look out for it. Tear off the thin, rubbery sheets, being careful to leave behind the part that is clinging to the rock.

Laverbread and Potato Cakes

300g (10oz) cold, boiled potatoes
125g (4oz) laverbread
4 spring onions, finely chopped
10ml (2 teaspoons) malt vinegar
1 egg yolk
freshly ground black pepper
60ml (4 tablespoons) wholewheat flour
40g (1½oz) butter, or, 90ml (6 tablespoons) melted bacon fat

Mash the potatoes to a smooth purée and mix in the laverbread, onions, vinegar, egg yolks and pepper. Form the mixture into eight small, round cakes, about 1 cm (½ inch) thick. Coat them in the flour.

Fry them in the butter or bacon fat until they are brown on both sides. Serve them very hot.

They are good with eggs and bacon. Serves 4.

Laverbread with Oats and Bacon

This savoury mixture is good with wholewheat bread and butter for lunch or supper.

40g (1½oz) butter
2 medium onions, thinly sliced
125g (4oz) rolled oats
225g (8oz) bacon, finely chopped
450g (1lb) laverbread

Melt the butter in a frying pan on a low heat. Mix in the onions and cook them until they are beginning to soften. Raise the heat and mix in the oats and bacon. Stir them around for 3 minutes so the oats brown. Lower the heat again and mix in the laverbread. Heat it through, stirring and mixing all the time. Serve hot. Serves 4.

Laverbread

Laver bread is the name given to laver when it has been pre-cooked and prepared for use as a base for other dishes.

The first thing that you must do with freshly gathered laver is wash it well, using at least four changes of water, to remove all the sand and grit. This is absolutely necessary since a gritty laverbread will ruin any dish that you make with it.

After washing, gently boil the laver in water to cover until it is tender and reduced to a thick, green mush. This will take about 6 hours. Then mince it and put it into plastic containers.

Laverbread will keep for up to 10 days in a cool place.

Laverbread Salad

Although the flavour of laver is less strong than that of dulse, it is still very distinctive, so keep any recipe made with it very simple, like this first course.

350g (12oz) laverbread
1 small onion, finely chopped
60ml (4 tablespoons) olive oil
juice ½ lemon
freshly ground black pepper
4 thin slices lemon

Put the laverbread into a bowl and mix it with the rest of the ingredients except the lemon. Divide the salad between four small dishes and top each one with a slice of lemon, made into a twist.

Serve the salads with wholewheat bread or toast and provide both a knife and a small spoon to eat it with. Serves 4.

Medicinal

Hand Gel

The green jelly that collects around the parts of the mincer after you have made the laverbread can be used as a hand gel and, if used regularly, will keep your hands exceptionally smooth and soft.

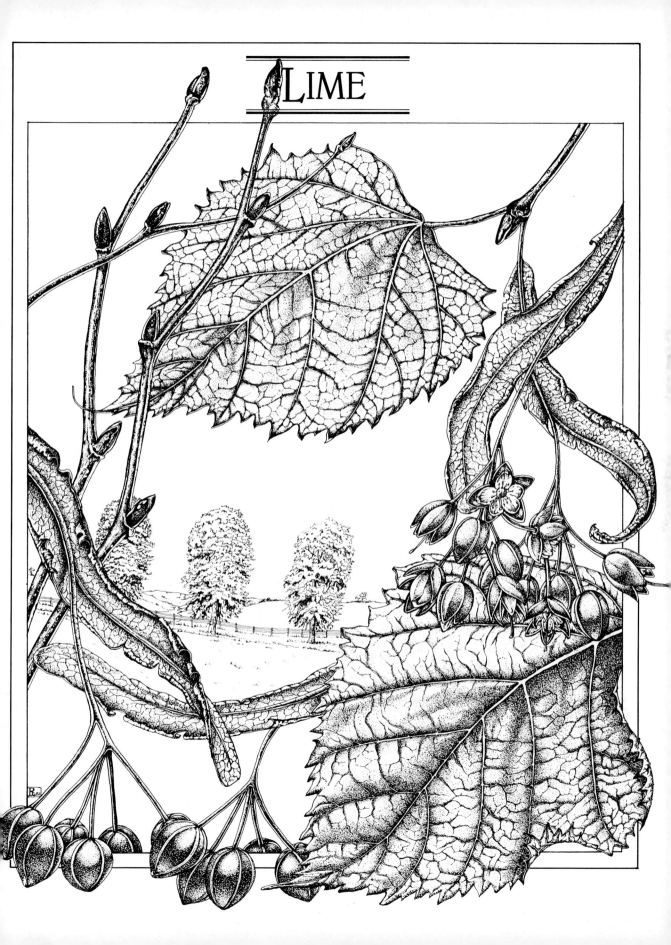

LIME

Availability

The lime tree grows throughout the northern temperate zone, particularly in Britain and Europe, but it can also be found in the United States. More common in the eastern states is Basswood (Tilea americana) which can be used in the same ways. In Australia it is grown in the cooler areas only.

Lime trees can be found growing along country lanes and in copses. Many have been artificially planted in parks and ornamental woods and by roadsides.

The young, bright green leaves are best picked as soon as they first appear (May in the northern hemisphere/November in Australasia) as then they are softer and have a better flavour.

The yellow green blossoms are usually ready for picking one and a half to two months later (early July in the northern hemisphere). Cut them from the twigs with scissors.

To dry lime blossoms

Spread them out on cardboard or on a wire rack that you have covered with muslin. Put them into the airing cupboard, a warm, airy room or a warming oven until they are dry and brittle. Keep them whole and store them in a light-tight container.

Tilleul (Lime Flower Tea)

This has a delicious honeyed flavour even if you do not sweeten it. Infuse 15 ml (1 tablespoon) dried lime flowers in 275 ml (½ pint) water for 4 minutes. Strain it and sweeten it if liked with honey.

Lime Leaf and Lemon Sandwiches

25 g (1 oz) lime leaves
juice ½ lemon
60 ml (4 tablespoons) olive oil
1 clove garlic, crushed with a pinch sea salt
freshly ground black pepper

Finely chop the lime leaves, mix them with the rest of the ingredients and leave them for 30 minutes.

Sandwich the mixture between slices of un-buttered wholewheat bread. Makes 2 rounds.

Lime Leaf and Tomato Sandwiches

Make these as lemon sandwiches, putting slices of tomato on top of the lemon filling. You may find these need butter.

Lime Leaf and Cheese Sandwiches

Make these as for lemon sandwiches, putting grated Cheddar cheese on top of the lemon filling.

Lime Leaf and Soured Cream Sandwiches

25 g (1 oz) lime leaves
60 ml (4 tablespoons) soured cream
10 ml (2 teaspoons) lemon juice
45 ml (3 tablespoons) chopped chives
freshly ground black pepper

Finely chop the lime leaves. Mix them with the rest of the ingredients and leave them for 30 minutes.

Sandwich the mixture between slices of un-buttered wholewheat bread. Makes 2 rounds.

Lime Leaf and Egg Sandwiches

Use half the amount of the soured cream filling and top it with slices of hardboiled egg. Use butter for these.

Medicinal

For hysteria, nervousness, palpitations, nervous headaches, migraines: Infuse 1 tablespoon dried lime flowers in 225 ml (8 fl oz) boiling water for 5 minutes. Strain and sweeten if liked with honey. Drink the whole amount three times a day.

To calm nervous and excited children: Boil 200 g (7 oz) lime flowers in 2 litres (3½ pints) water for 10 minutes. Strain and add to the bath water for a soothing bath.

To clear the skin of impurities: Boil 50 g (2 oz) dried lime flowers in 1 litre (1¾ pints) water for 20 minutes. Strain and cool and use daily as a skin lotion. It also helps to combat wrinkles.

LATE SUMMER

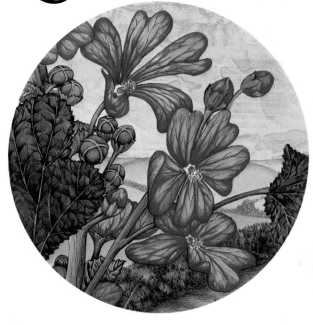

ANGELICA

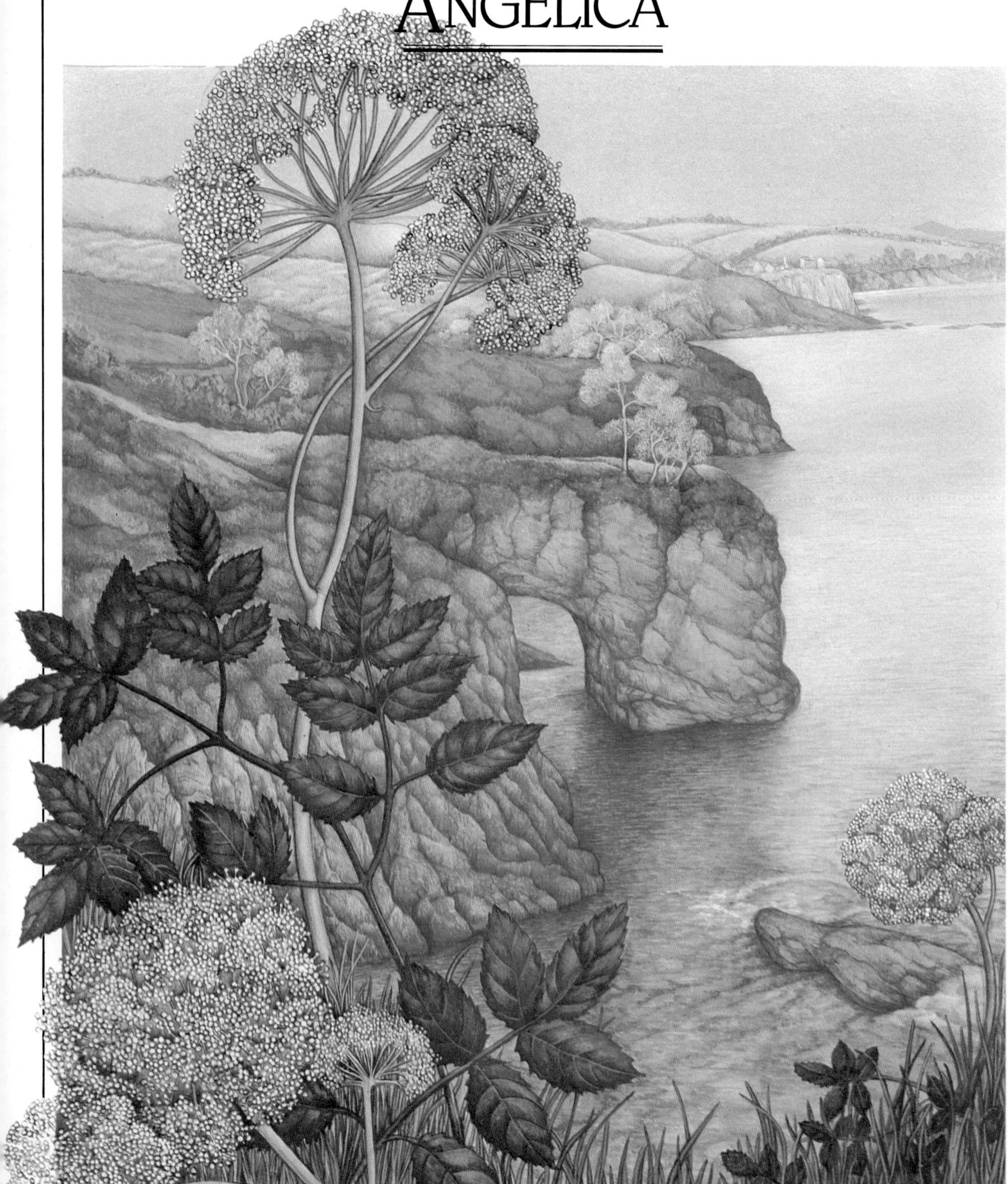

Availability

Angelica grows wild in most northern countries of Europe and also in the Pyrenees. It is common in Scotland, but more scarce in the southern part of Britain. In the United States it is also a plant of the most northern areas.

When angelica grows wild it loves damp, moist soil and it can often be found in moist woods, by mountain streams and in coastal regions. It may also be found as a garden escape in drier, more unlikely areas. In Australia it is only found in cultivation.

The leaves and stems of angelica appear early in the spring. The leaves can be used from then until autumn (late September in the northern hemisphere/March in Australasia), but the stems are best used in late summer (July to August in the northern hemisphere/January to February in Australasia) when they have grown fairly large but are still tender and without any stringy fibres. The flowers appear at the same time and the seeds can be collected in early autumn.

Cut both leaves and stems from the plant with scissors. They are best used fresh but the leaves can be kept in a plastic bag in the bottom of the refrigerator for up to two days. The seed heads should be cut off with a 15 cm (6 inch) piece of stalk attached and hung up to dry in a paper bag.

If you do not need the seeds, and you are able to watch over a particular plant, cut off the flowering head as soon as it appears. This will make the leaves stay usable for a longer time.

If the roots are required for medicinal purposes, dig them in the autumn and dry them like dandelion roots (see dandelion entry). When dried, they should be grey-brown and wrinkled on the outside and spongy white on the inside.

Candied Angelica Stems

Use candied angelica to decorate cakes, ice creams, mousses and trifles. Only candy the tenderest bright green stalks.

A sugar (candy) thermometer is a great help when candying.

225 g (8 oz) angelica stalks
450 g (1 lb) sugar
575 ml (1 pint) water
50 g (2 oz) icing (confectioner's) sugar

Cut the angelica stalks into 10 cm (4 inch) lengths. Put them into boiling water and cook them for 7–10 minutes, so they are just beginning to become pliable. Drain them and refresh them in cold water. Drain them again and peel away any stringy fibres. Put the stalks into a shallow dish.

Put the sugar and water into a saucepan and stir on a low heat until the sugar dissolves; bring to the boil and pour the boiling syrup over the angelica stems. Cover them and leave them for 24 hours.

Repeat this boiling twice more. Then on the fourth day heat the syrup to 120 C/245 F. Put in the angelica and bring it to the boil. Take the pan from the heat and let the bubbles subside. Bring the syrup to the boil again and remove. Repeat this twice more and then cool completely with the angelica still in the syrup.

Lift out the angelica stalks and put them on a wire rack to dry. Coat each piece in icing sugar and put them onto a non-stick baking sheet. Put them into a preheated Reg ¼/100C/225F oven until completely dried (30 minutes–1 hour, depending on the thickness of the stems). They should be dry and not sticky.

Cool the candied stems on a wire rack and then wrap them in waxed paper. Store them in an airtight container. They will keep for up to a year.

Prawns in Angelica Mayonnaise

The flavour of fresh lime juice goes so well with angelica that it is used in the following two recipes. Lemon juice can be used instead if limes are not available.

Angelica goes superbly with sea-food.

350 (12oz) prawns or shrimps, unshelled
60 ml (4 tablespoons) mayonnaise
15 ml (1 tablespoon) chopped angelica leaves
  (young ones)
pinch curry powder
30 ml (2 tablespoons) fresh lime juice

Mix together the mayonnaise, angelica leaves, curry powder and lime juice. Fold in the prawns or shrimps.

Serve the prawns or shrimps as a first course for six, or with a selection of salads as a main meal for four.

Cod baked with Angelica and Tomatoes

675–900 g (1½–2lb) cod fillet, cut into 8 even sized
    pieces
pinch cayenne pepper
grated rind and juice 1 lime
60 ml (4 tablespoons) olive oil
1 medium onion, finely chopped
350 g (12 oz) tomatoes, scalded, skinned and chopped

Heat the oven to Reg 6/200C/400F. Put the pieces
of cod into a large, flat, ovenproof dish and scatter
them with the angelica, cayenne pepper and lime
rind.

Beat the lime juice and oil together and pour
them over the cod. Scatter the onion and tomatoes
on top.

Cover the dish with foil and put it into the oven
for 25 minutes. Serve the cod, straight from the
dish, with the juices spooned over it. Serves 4.

Angelica with Tart Fruits

If a large sprig of angelica is cooked with tart fruits
such as apples or rhubarb, it gives them a mellow,
scented flavour. Use it for plain stewed fruits, fruit
compotes and fruit purées for making into more
complicated dishes such as mousses and fruit
fools.

Apple and Angelica Snow

Although this recipe includes gelatin, the mixture
does not set firm like a mousse since yoghurt is
used instead of whipped cream. It is more like a
thick, pale green cloud, and it makes a very
refreshing sweet.

675 g (1½ lbs) cooking apples
1 large angelica sprig
4 cloves
150 ml (¼ pint) dry cider
15 g (½ oz) gelatin
100 g (3½ oz) honey
2 eggs, separated
150 ml (¼ pint) natural yoghurt
candied angelica stems for decoration (optional)

Core and chop the apples. There is no need to peel
them. Put them into a saucepan with the angelica
and cloves and 100 ml (3½ fl oz) cider. Cover them
and set them on a low heat for about 15 minutes so
they can be beaten to a purée. Rub them through a
sieve.

In a small pan, soak the gelatin in the remaining
cider. Return the apple purée to the cleaned
saucepan. Set it on a low heat. Add the honey and

stir until it dissolves. Beat in the egg yolks, one at a
time, making sure the apples do not boil. Gently
melt the gelatin and stir it into the apple mixture.
Take the pan from the heat and cool the mixture
until it is on the point of setting.

Stir the yoghurt into the mixture. Stiffly whip
the egg whites and fold them in with a metal
spoon. Pour the snow into a bowl and leave it in a
cool place for two hours to set. Just before
serving, decorate the top with thin sticks of
candied angelica. Serves 4–6.

Medicinal

A strengthening tonic: Infuse 15 ml (a tablespoon) chopped angelica leaves in 275 ml (½ pint)
boiling water for 10 minutes. Strain. Drink the
whole amount every day. This is a favourite drink
in Finland.

For hoarseness and sore throat: Boil 25 g (1 oz)
bruised angelica root in 1.15 l (2 pints) water for
three hours. Strain and add 255 g (8 oz) honey.
Take two tablespoons every night and morning
and twice during the day.

For feverish colds: Make up the infusion as for the
tonic. Add the juice of half a lemon and honey to
taste. Drink it several times a day.

To relieve flatulence: Chew angelica stems.
Or, infuse 25 g (1 oz) bruised dried angelica root in
575 ml (1 pint) boiling water for 15 minutes.
Strain and drink 30 ml (2 tablespoons) four times a
day. This is also good for indigestion.
Or, boil 5 ml (1 teaspoon) chopped fresh root in
225 ml (8 fl oz) water for 1 minute. Strain. Take
the whole amount twice a day.

BLACKBERRY

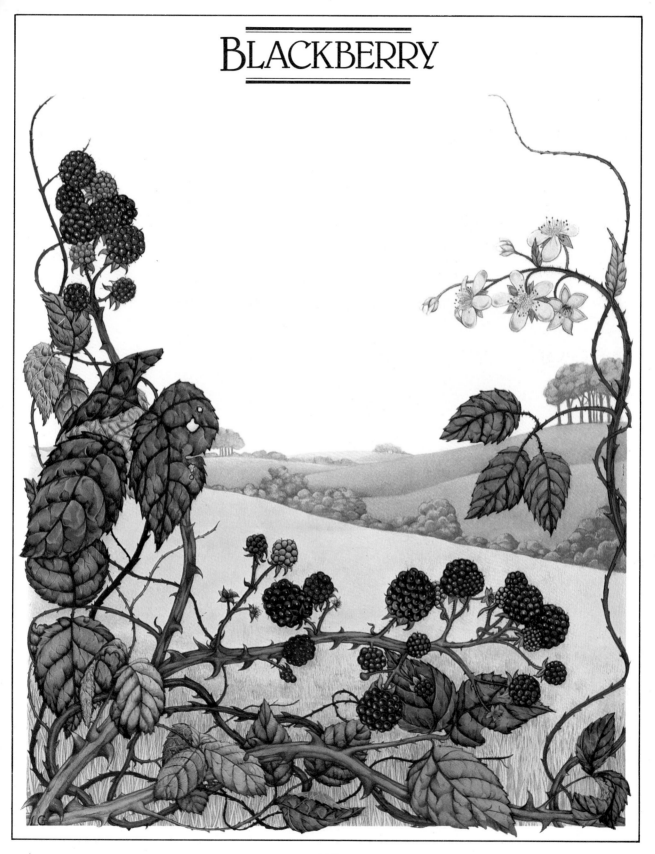

Availability

The blackberry grows extensively throughout North America, the British Isles, Europe, Australia and New Zealand. It rapidly spreads in woods, hedges, heaths and waste places. The berries, which are the part most commonly used, are ready for picking in late summer (late August in the northern hemisphere) and their season usually lasts until the middle of October (April in Australasia). The large berries on the ends of the clusters are the ones that ripen first and these are generally the sweetest and juiciest.

Upside-down Blackberry and Apple Cake

125 g (4 oz) butter
125 g (4 oz) honey plus
30 ml (2 tablespoons) melted honey
125 g (4 oz) wholewheat flour
5 ml (1 teaspoon) baking powder
2 eggs, beaten
butter for greasing
225 g (8 oz) blackberries
2 large eating apples

Heat the oven to Reg 4/180C/350F/. Beat the butter until it is light and fluffy. Beat in the 125 g (4 oz) honey. Mix the flour with the baking powder and beat them into the butter and honey alternately with the eggs. Butter a 20 cm (8 inch) diameter cake tin. Put in the blackberries. Peel, core and finely chop the apples and mix them with the blackberries. Spoon the melted honey over them. Cover the blackberries and apples evenly with cake mixture. Bake the cake for 25 minutes or until the top is golden brown. Turn it out onto a round, flat plate and serve it hot with thin cream.

Blackberry Tremble

675 g (1½ lbs) blackberries
30 ml (2 tablespoons) water
4 cloves
2 allspice berries
30 ml (2 tablespoons) light brown (demerara) sugar
10 ml (2 teaspoons) arrowroot

Put the blackberries into a saucepan with the water, cloves and allspice and cook them on a low heat until they are soft and juicy (about 15 minutes). Rub them through a sieve and return them to the rinsed out pan. Stir in the sugar and keep the purée on a low heat until the sugar dissolves. Put the arrowroot into a bowl and gradually mix in 90 ml (6 tablespoons) blackberry purée. When you have a smooth paste, stir it back into the saucepan. Bring the purée to the boil, stirring, and let it bubble gently for about 3 minutes so it is thick but transparent. Pour the mixture into a serving bowl and put it into a cool place so it becomes just set and slightly trembly.

Blackberry Pudding

675 g (1½ lbs) blackberries
75 g (3 oz) honey
1 loaf day old granary or wholewheat bread

Put the blackberries with the honey into a saucepan and cook them on a low heat until the juice begins to run and the honey is melted (about 5 minutes). Cut the bread into 1 cm (⅜ inch) thick slices and remove the crusts. Cut one slice to fit the bottom of an 850 ml (1½ pint) pudding basin. Cut some into wedge shapes and overlap them round the sides of the basin so they line it completely. Pour in the blackberries and cover them completely with more slices of bread. Cover the basin with a flat plate and put a weight on top. Put the pudding into the refrigerator for at least 12 hours so the bread becomes soaked in the syrup. Serve with natural yoghurt or soured cream.

Blackberry Jam

2 kg (4 lbs) blackberries
120 ml (8 tablespoons) water
2 kg (4 lbs) sugar
juice 1 lemon

Put the blackberries into a preserving pan with the water and cook them on a low heat until they are soft and juicy. Warm the sugar in a low oven and stir it into the blackberries. Add the lemon juice. Stir on a low heat until the sugar is dissolved. Then raise the heat and boil until setting point is reached (about 15 minutes). Pour the jam into hot jars and cover it with wax paper. Cover it completely when cold.

Wine and Cordials

Blackberry Vinegar

675 g (1½ lbs) blackberries (picked in three batches)
one 369 ml (13 fl oz) bottle of white wine vinegar
enough honey to equal weight of strained vinegar
 (about 225–350 g [8–12 oz])

Put 225 g (8 oz) blackberries into a bowl with the vinegar. Cover and leave them for 4 days in a cool place. Strain the vinegar and put it back into the bowl with a further 225 g (8 oz) blackberries. Leave for four more days, and repeat the process. Strain the vinegar through a jelly bag and weigh it. Put it into a saucepan with the appropriate amount of honey. Stir until the honey has dissolved and bring the vinegar to the boil on a low heat. Boil for 5 minutes and skim well. Pour the vinegar into an earthenware jug and cover it with a linen tea cloth, folded into four. Tie the cloth down securely and leave the vinegar for 24 hours. Pour it back into the rinsed-out vinegar bottle. There should be an equal volume of blackberry vinegar as there was white wine vinegar in the beginning. Use the blackberry vinegar, diluted with hot or cold water, as a refreshing drink.

Blackberry Wine

for 4.6 litres (1 gallon):

1.35 kg (3 lbs) blackberries
225 g (8 oz) raisins, chopped
1.8 kg (4 lbs) sugar
4.6 litres (1 gallon) water
Bordeaux yeast
yeast nutrient
pectolase

Wash the blackberries, put them into a plastic container and pound them until they are well mashed. Add the raisins and the sugar. Bring the water to the boil and pour it over the blackberries, raisins and sugar. Cool and add the yeast, yeast nutrient and pectolase. Leave for 5 days, stirring twice a day. Strain the wine into a 4.6 litre (1 gallon) jar and fit a fermentation lock. Rack the wine until it is clear. Bottle it, and leave it for 6 months before opening. The wine will be very dark and rich, in fact like a good Bordeaux.

Medicinal

For diarrhœa and similar complaints

either:

1 blackberry root
water

Peel the bark from the root and dry it in a low oven or the hot sun. Put 25 g (1 oz) of the dried bark into a saucepan with 850 ml (1½ pints) water. Boil until the liquid is reduced to 1 pint and strain. Cool and take a teacupful every 1½ hours. (The root should be lifted in the autumn. The dried bark will keep for a year for use when needed.)

or

25 g (1 oz) dried blackberry leaves
575 ml (1 pint) boiling water

Put the leaves into a jug and pour the boiling water over them. Strain and cool the liquid and take a teacupful every 2 hours.

Scratches and scalds: For scratches received while picking blackberries and other minor cuts and abrasions. It is also useful for minor scalds. Crush a handful of blackberry leaves and rub them on the scratch to ease the pain and stop the bleeding.

Blackberry Syrup

For coughs, colds, bronchial catarrh, sore throat:

2 kg (5 lbs) blackberries
1 cinnamon stick about 15 cm (6 inches) long
120 ml (8 tablespoons) water
675 g (1½ lbs) honey

Put the blackberries into a large saucepan or a preserving pan with the cinnamon stick and water. Set them on a low heat and cook them until they are soft and juicy (about 15 minutes). Strain the blackberries through muslin to extract the juice. Return the juice to the rinsed-out pan and stir in the sugar or honey. When it has dissolved, boil the juice for 10 minutes. Pour the syrup into hot, sterilised jars and cork it straight away. As a remedy, take 15 ml (1 tablespoon) in a glass of hot or cold water every 2 hours.

ASH

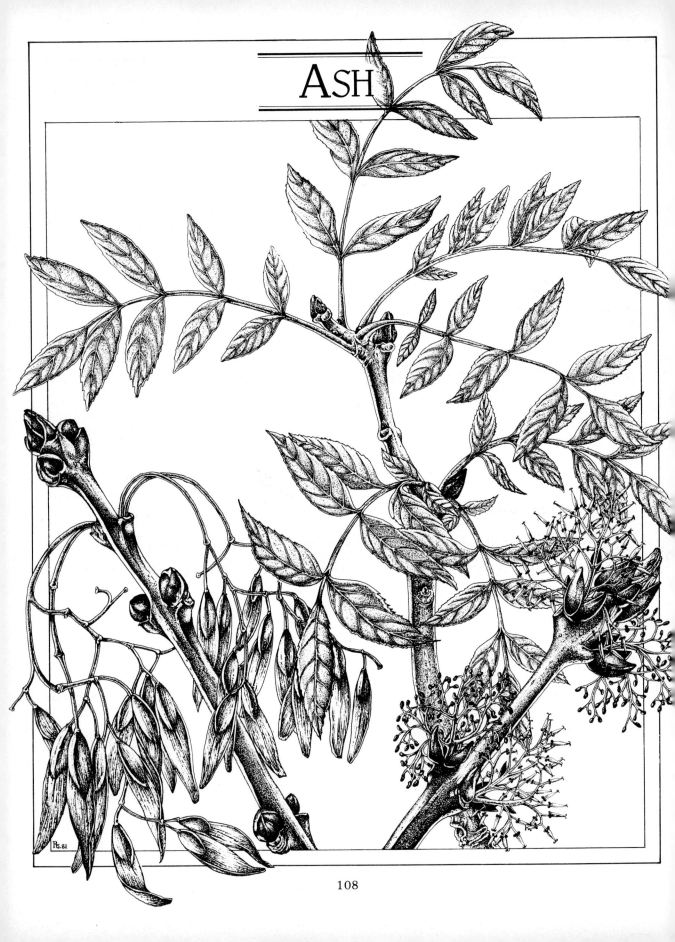

Availability

The ash tree is common throughout Britain, Scandinavia and Europe. There are three related species in the United States, Fraxinus americana, Fraxinus pennsylvania and Fraxinus oregona. These can all be used in the same ways. The ash is extensively grown in Australia but not so much a wild plant.

Ash trees grow in woods and along hedge-rows and some are free standing in parks and fields. The keys for pickling should be picked from mid to late summer (July in the northern hemisphere/ January in Australasia), when they are small, green and crisp textured and in no way tough or stringy.

The bark and leaves are used medicinally. The best bark is that taken from the root, but in spring it may also be taken from the branches. The leaves should be picked in early summer when they are slightly sticky. They can be dried and powdered and kept in air tight containers.

Pickled Ash Keys

This pickle goes particularly well with strong cheese and cold meats.

125 g (4 oz) ash keys
15 ml (1 tablespoon) grated horseradish
5 ml (1 teaspoon) black peppercorns
425 ml (¾ pint) cider vinegar
150 ml (¼ pint) dry cider
30 ml (2 tablespoons) honey

Put the ash keys into cold water, bring them to the boil and boil them for 5 minutes. Drain them, put them into cold water again and repeat the process. They should be quite tender and not at all bitter.

Pack the keys into a 450 g (1 lb) jar, scattering in the horseradish and a few black peppercorns as you go.

Put the vinegar, cider and honey into a saucepan and stir on a low heat for the honey to dissolve. Bring them to the boil and pour them into the jar of ash keys. Wait for about 10 minutes for the liquid to settle and top it up again. Wait and top up once more.

Lightly cover the jars and put them into a preheated Reg under ¼/100C/200F oven for 1 hour. Take them out and seal them tightly. Leave the pickle for two weeks before opening.

Medicinal

For facial neuralgia: Infuse 45 ml (3 tablespons) chopped dried ash leaves in 1 litre (1¾ pints) boiling water for 15 minutes. Strain. Sweeten only slightly with honey. Drink a cupful three times a day before meals.

For gout and rheumatism: Infuse 25 g (1 oz) fresh leaves and 6 mint leaves in 1 litre (1¾ pints) boiling water for 15 minutes. Strain. Drink 1 cupful every three hours during attacks.

A mild laxative: Infuse 25 g (1 oz) chopped fresh leaves (or 15 g (½ oz) dried) in 575 ml (1 pint) boiling water for 20 minutes. Strain and take 150 ml (¼ pint) four times a day.

For fevers: Make a decoction by boiling 25 g (1 oz) bark in 1 litre (1¾ pints) water for 5 minutes. Strain and take 1 cupful three times a day before meals.

Veterinary

Encourage all farm stock to eat ash leaves as they are tonic and mildly laxative.
For fevers, let them feed off the leaves.
In cases of rheumatism, give several handfuls of chopped ash leaves every day in a bran mash.
For internal wind, boil 10 ash keys in 275 ml (½ pint) mixed milk and water for 5 minutes. Strain the decoction and give it to the animal to drink.

CHAMOMILE

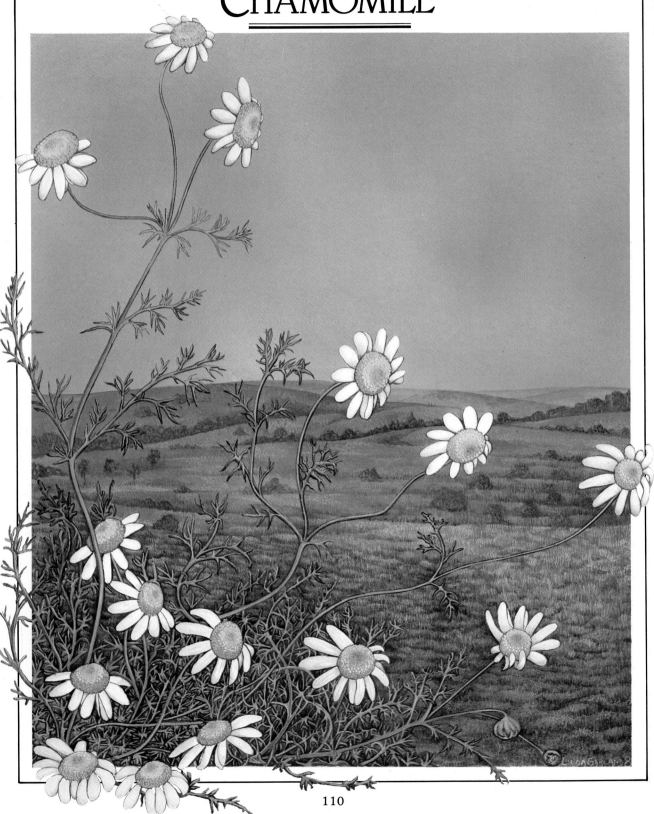

Availability

Chamomile grows throughout France and Germany and the southern part of Britain. It is not found wild in the United States but is often cultivated.

Chamomile is mainly to be found on dry heaths and grassland and it favours sandy soil. In some places it will spread to form a carpet which smells very sweet whenever it is walked over.

Pick chamomile flowers throughout the latter part of summer (July to September in the northern hemisphere/January to March in Australasia). Cut off the small flower heads with scissors and either use them fresh as soon as possible or spread them on muslin covered racks to dry.

Sherry and Chamomile Punch

In some parts of Spain chamomile is used to flavour sherry. Together they make a warming, flowery tasting punch that can be served as a winter aperitif.

1½ lemons
15 ml (1 tablespoon) dried chamomile flowers
275 ml (½ pint) boiling water
275 ml (½ pint) medium dry sherry
15 ml (1 tablespoon) honey

Thinly slice one lemon and put it into a jug with the chamomile. Pour the boiling water over them and leave them to infuse for 10 minutes. Strain.

Put the sherry and honey into a saucepan. Heat them to simmering point, stirring. Pour them into the infusion. Pour the punch into four glasses and put a thin slice of lemon into each one.

Chamomile Tea

Infuse 15 ml (1 tablespoon) dried chamomile flowers in 275 ml (½ pint) boiling water for 10 minutes. It is important to always cover chamomile when making an infusion. Strain and sweeten with honey to taste.

Chamomile tea is the brew that made Peter Rabbit hide under the bedclothes! In actual fact it tastes very pleasant. Drink it as a calming mid-morning drink instead of coffee; or as a soothing nightcap.

In summer the tea can be left to become quite cold after sweetening and it makes a refreshing and thirst quenching drink.

Medicinal

To bring out highlights in blonde hair: Infuse 50 g (2 oz) dried chamomile flowers in 1.5 litres (2¼ pints) boiling water for 15 minutes. Strain and use the infusion as the final rinse after washing the hair.

A lotion for oily skin: Infuse 15 ml (1 tablespoon) each dried chamomile and yarrow in 275 ml (½ pint) boiling water for 15 minutes. Strain and bottle. Use the infusion to wash the face every morning, letting it dry on the skin.

To sooth teething babies: Infuse 15 g (½ oz) dried chamomile flowers in 575 ml (1 pint) boiling water for 10 minutes. Stir and give in doses of 5 ml (1 teaspoon).

For hysteria, nervousness and insomnia: Infuse 25 g (1 oz) dried chamomile in 575 ml (1 pint) boiling water for 10 minutes. Strain. Take the infusion frequently in amounts of about 150 ml (¼ pint). For insomnia, take as the last drink of the day on going to bed.

Chamomile rub: Put 50 g (2 oz) dried chamomile flowers into a saucepan with 500 ml (15 fl oz) olive oil. Heat it gently for 2 hours, covered. Strain the oil and bottle it.

For rheumatism and gout, rub the oil on the aching limb.

For sprains, apply a compress soaked in oil. Keep it in place with a bandage and change it every three hours.

PARASOL MUSHROOM

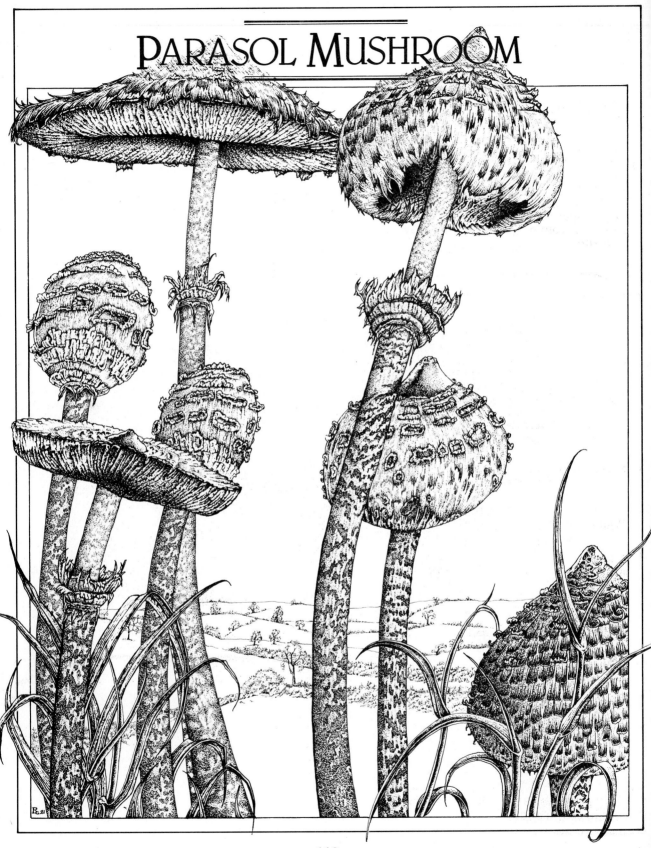

Availability

The parasol mushroom grows throughout Britain, Europe and Scandinavia and in the central, southern, south-eastern and north-eastern states of America. In Australia the slender parasol mushroom or Lepiota gracilenta is the variety found. It is edible when young, but is uncommon.

It grows in grassy pastures and meadows, in orchards, on the edges of woodland, in woodland clearings, by roadsides and on railway banks. If you are lucky, you may even find one growing on the back lawn. Available throughout summer (April to August in the northern hemisphere). Parasol mushrooms often grow in groups and sometimes can be found in perfect "fairy rings".

Parasol mushrooms start off with a drum-stick stipe and a closed, egg-shaped cap. They are best picked just as the cap has flattened but before it begins to turn up slightly at the edges. Twist or cut them from the ground. They will keep for up to 24 hours in a cool, dry place. After this, they begin to take on a rusty tinge and the flavour becomes stronger.

Cooking Parasol Mushrooms

Parasol mushrooms are often very large and can be up to 25 cm (10 inches) in diameter. One can often weigh 175–225 g (6–8 oz) and will be sufficient to feed four people. There is no need to peel a parasol mushroom but check around the top of the stipe for insects.

To cook a parasol mushroom for breakfast, cut it into triangular wedges as you would a cake. Brown them quickly in hot fat or dripping, under side down first. They are superb with bacon and eggs.

To make them a special breakfast feature, serve the mushroom wedges on fried bread which you have spread with a little tomato purée and sprinkled very lightly with cayenne pepper.

Fried Rice with Parasol Mushrooms

This makes a tasty all-in-one meal. Stir-fried vegetables are a good accompaniment.

300 g (10 oz) long grain brown rice
175 g (6 oz) parasol mushrooms
225 g (8 oz) cooked lean ham
2 eggs
60 ml (4 tablespoons) tamari or soy sauce
90 ml (3 fl oz) sunflower oil

Boil the rice in lightly salted water until tender. Drain it, refresh it with cold water and drain it again. Cut the parasol mushroom into 2.5 cm (1 inch) squares. Finely chop the ham. Beat the eggs with the tamari or soy sauce.

Heat 60 ml (4 tablespoons) of the oil in a large frying pan on a high heat. Put in the pieces of mushroom and brown them quickly on both sides. Remove them. Do this in two batches if necessary.

Put in the remaining oil. Mix in the rice and ham. Pour in the egg mixture and fork everything around until the rice grains have a fluffy, set coating. Mix the mushrooms back into the pan, heat them through quickly and serve. Serves 4.

Parasol Mushrooms with Bacon

Half a large mushroom with a topping of bacon can make a satisfying meal.

2 parasol mushrooms, each 18–20 cm (7–8 inches) in diameter
450 g (1 lb) smoked bacon
up to 45 g (3 oz) butter
60 ml (4 tablespoons) Worcestershire sauce
60 ml (4 tablespoons) chopped parsley

Remove the stalks from the mushrooms. Cut each mushroom in half. Finely chop the bacon.

Melt 25 g (1 oz) of the butter in a large frying pan on a low heat. Put in the bacon and cook it until it browns, stirring frequently. Remove it and drain it on absorbent paper towels.

Raise the heat under the pan slightly. Put in one or two mushroom halves, depending on the size of the pan, and brown them on both sides. Remove them and keep them warm. Cook the remaining mushroom halves in the same way, adding more butter if necessary. Put them with the first halves, on a large serving plate, bottom up.

Return all the bacon pieces to the pan. Add the parsley. Pour in the sauce and let it bubble. Take the pan from the heat and spoon the bacon, parsley and sauce over the mushrooms. Serves 4.

CORN AND WATER MINT

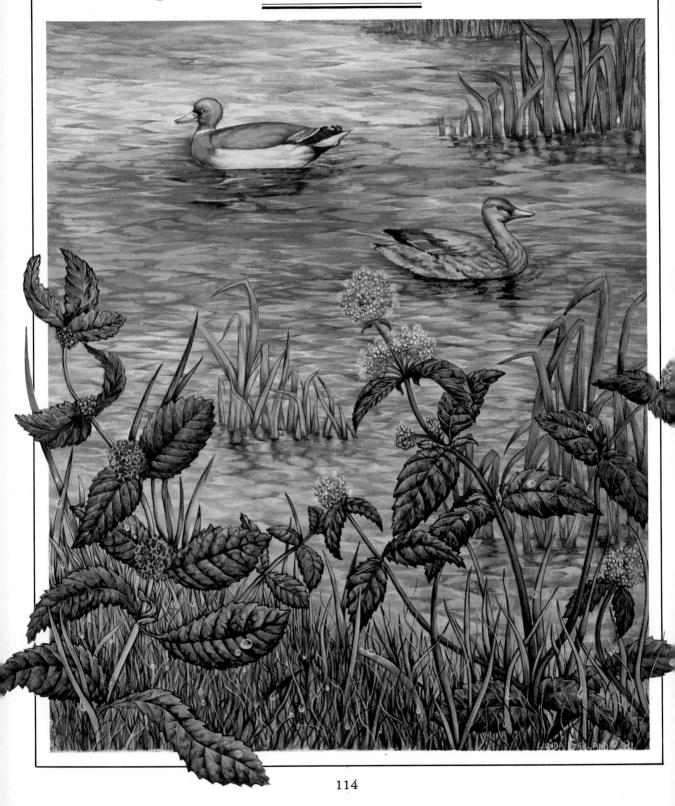

CORN MINT   MENTHA ARVENSIS
WATER MINT   MENTHA AQUATICA
Local Names: Corn Mint: Apple Mint, Lamb's Tongue.
Water Mint: Bishopsweed, Bishopswort, Horse Mint,
Lilac Flower, Marsh Mint, Wild Mint.

Availability

Both mints grow throughout Britain, Europe and Scandinavia. Corn mint can be found all over north America, and the American Wild Mint, Mentha canadensis, which has a slightly similar flavour to water mint, can be found from New Brunswick and Virginia, west to the Pacific coast.

Corn mint grows mainly on arable farm land and heath land, in woodland clearings and along woodland rides.

Water mint loves wet places. It can be found along the banks of rivers and streams, in water-meadows and marshes and in damp woodland. The American wild mint grows in similar places.

Corn mint flowers from mid summer until autumn and water mint from late summer to autumn. The leaves of both can be used all through summer and autumn (June to September in the northern hemisphere/December to March in Australasia).

Spearmint (Mentha shicata) is the most common in Australia, and grows in damp areas.

If you only need a few leaves, pick them from the stems by hand. If more are required, cut the whole stems with scissors. They will keep fresh for several days if they are put into a jar of water.

Cucumber, Walnut and Mint Salad

Serve this salad as a first course. Mint and coriander give a fresh spiciness to the dressing.

2 small ridge cucumbers
125 g (4 oz) chopped walnuts
45 ml (3 tablespoons) corn or water mint
90 ml (6 tablespoons) natural yoghurt
1 clove garlic, crushed with a pinch sea salt
2.5 ml (½ teaspoon) ground coriander
4 mint leaves

Cut the cucumbers in half lengthways. Discard the seeds and chop the rest. Put the cucumber into a bowl with the walnuts and mint.

Beat together the remaining ingredients and fold them into the salad. Divide the salad between four small bowls and garnish each one with a mint leaf. Serves 4.

Spiced Minted Lamb

Mint and lamb are the perfect partners, be it a traditional roast and mint sauce or something spicier.

one half shoulder of lamb
150 ml (¼ pint) natural yoghurt
30 ml (2 tablespoons) corn mint
5 ml (1 teaspoon) cumin seeds
5 ml (1 teaspoon) ground coriander
1 clove garlic, crushed with a pinch sea salt

Heat the oven to Reg 6/200 C/400 F. Bone the lamb. Mix the remaining ingredients together.

Spoon half the yoghurt mixture over the cut surface of the lamb. Roll up the lamb and tie it with fine cotton string. Put it into a casserole and spoon the remaining yoghurt mixture on top.

Cover the casserole and put it into the oven for 1 hour 15 minutes.

Take out the lamb, carve it and arrange it on a warm serving dish. Skim the juices in the casserole and spoon them over the lamb. Serves 4.

Plum and Mint Jelly

Serve this jelly with roast lamb or game.

1.35 kg (3 lbs) dark cooking plums
426 ml (¾ pint) water
150 ml (¼ pint) red wine vinegar
225 g (8 oz) light brown (demerara) sugar
  to every 275 ml (½ pint) juice
90 ml (6 tablespoons) very finely chopped water mint

Wipe the plums. With a sharp knife, slit each one all round. Put the plums into a preserving pan with the water and vinegar. Bring them to the boil and simmer them gently for 45 minutes so they are very soft, turning them occasionally. Mash them down as they soften. Remove any stones that come to the surface.

Strain the plums through a scalded jelly bag and leave them to drip until all the juice is through the bag (about 2 hours). Measure the juice. Weigh the appropriate amount of sugar and warm it in a low oven.

Put the juice into the cleaned pan and bring it to the boil. Add the sugar and stir until it dissolves. Bring the juice to the boil and boil until it reaches setting point.

Take the pan from the heat and stir in the mint. Cool the jelly to lukewarm and stir it again to distribute the mint evenly. Pour it into warm pots. Cover it with waxed paper circles. Let it get quite cold and cover it with cellophane circles or lids. Makes about 350g (12oz).

Mint and Chocolate Ice Cream

This ice cream has a creamy chocolate flavour with a delicate suggestion of mint. Use water mint for the fresher flavour.

50g (2oz) water mint leaves
75g (3oz) honey
125ml (4floz) water
juice ½ lemon
3 egg yolks
725ml (1¼ pints) thin cream
100g (3½oz) dark chocolate

Put the mint leaves, honey and water into a saucepan and set them on a low heat, stirring until the honey dissolves. Bring them to the boil and boil for 5 minutes. Take the pan from the heat. Strain the syrup and add the lemon juice.

Beat the egg yolks until they are light and fluffy. Pour the syrup onto them and keep beating until the mixture is thick.

Break up the chocolate and put it into a saucepan with the cream. Set them on a low heat and stir until the chocolate has dissolved. Bring the mixture to just below boiling point, then take it from the heat and cool it. Whip it into the yolk mixture.

Chill the mixture and then pour it into a bowl or freezing tray. Put it into the coldest part of the freezer or into the ice compartment of the refrigerator, set at the lowest temperature. Freeze it to a slush (about 2 hours). Take it out, put it into a large bowl and whisk it.

Put the whisked ice cream into a plastic container, cover it and freeze it completely (about 3 hours). After this it can be taken into room temperature for 20 minutes and served; or it can be kept in the freezer for up to two months or the freezing compartment of the refrigerator (now back at normal setting) for up to 2 weeks. Serves 8.

Mint Sauce to Last the Winter

Once mint dies away there is nothing to serve with mutton or lamb until the next year, so store it, ready chopped, in vinegar.

125g (4oz) corn or water mint leaves
10ml (2 teaspoons) honey
about 150ml (¼pint) white wine vinegar

Finely chop the mint leaves and pack them tightly into a 450g (1lb) jar, putting 5ml (1 teaspoon) honey one third and two thirds of the way up.

Pour in a little vinegar and let it settle to the bottom. This may take about 15 minutes. Go on pouring in a little at a time and letting it sink until it covers the mint by about 3mm (⅛inch).

Cover the sauce and store it in a cool, dark place.

To prevent milk souring in hot weather

Have a bunch of corn mint in the dairy.

Medicinal

For a headache: Make mint vinegar. Put a large sprig of water mint into a bottle of cider vinegar. Put the cap on the bottle and leave the vinegar in a sunny window for 3 weeks. Change the sprig for a fresh one. The vinegar is now ready to use but will keep for up to a year.

To ease a headache, steep a cotton cloth in mint vinegar and lay it across the forehead, whilst relaxing, for 15 minutes.

For diarrhoea: Infuse 25g (1oz) dried water mint in 575ml (1pint) boiling water for 15 minutes. Strain, sweeten with honey and take frequently in wineglassful doses.

For colds and influenza: Infuse 15ml (1 tablespoon) dried or 30ml (2 tablespoons) fresh water mint in 250ml (8floz) boiling water for 10 minutes. Strain and sweeten with honey. Drink the whole amount as often as you please.

Veterinary

Feed mints to milking animals when there is too free a flow of milk or when it is necessary to dry the animal off before calving. Give two handfuls a day at milking time.
Do not feed mint to an animal when you wish to maintain or increase the milk supply.
A mint infusion added to the drinking water is a good tonic for bulls and stallions.

Availability

Chanterelle mushrooms grow throughout Britain, Europe, Scandinavia and the United States. They are one of the most popular of edible mushrooms and are frequently sold in markets and served in the world's top restaurants. They are not found in Australasia.

Chanterelles grow in established woodlands where there is a mixture of deciduous and conifer trees and where the woodland floor is covered with bracken. They seldom, however, grow where the trees are close together and the bracken thick, preferring wide, airy woodland paths and places where the trees are widely spaced. Once you have found them, return to the same spot every year for they are sure always to be there.

Chanterelles can be found from mid-summer to early autumn (late June to October in the northern hemisphere).

When picking chanterelles, it is best to cut them from the ground near the base of the stipe (stem). Twisting them out sometimes damages them. They stay fresh for a good twenty four hours after picking if they are spread out in a cool, dry place.

There is no need to peel chanterelles for cooking. They are seldom attacked by insects, but it is wise to check at the top of the stipe.

Cooking Chanterelles

Even if you can only find a few, it is worth picking chanterelles to make them into a side vegetable or garnish.

Thinly slice them and simmer them in butter [50g (2oz) to 225g (8oz)] on a low heat for 10 minutes. Season them with black pepper and add a squeeze of lemon juice. Serve them in small heaps beside the meat.

Eggs Baked with Chanterelle Mushrooms

225g (8oz) chanterelle mushrooms
60ml (4 tablespoons) chopped parsley
juice ½ lemon
8 eggs
150ml (¼ pint) soured cream

Heat the oven to Reg 6/200C/400F. Finely chop the mushrooms and scatter them evenly in the bottom of a large, flat, ovenproof dish. Scatter in the parsley and moisten them with the lemon juice.

Carefully break the eggs on top. Lightly beat the soured cream to make it smooth and spoon it over the eggs.

Cover the dish with buttered foil and put it into the oven for 20 minutes. The white should be set but the yolks still slightly liquid. Serve the eggs and mushrooms straight from the dish. Serves 4.

Chanterelles Simmered in Milk

Cooked in milk, chanterelles are excellent with chicken dishes or piled on buttered toast. To make them really rich and delicious, use half milk and half thick cream, and serve them on small rounds of toast as a first course.

175–225g (6–8oz) Chanterelle mushrooms
40g (1½oz) butter
150ml (¼ pint) milk
60ml (4 tablespoons) chopped parsley
freshly ground black pepper

Thinly slice the chanterelles. Melt the butter in a saucepan on a low heat. Stir in the chanterelles and cook them gently for 1 minute. Pour in the milk and parsley and plenty of pepper. Simmer gently, uncovered, for 15 minutes. Serves 4.

Chanterelle Scramble

Chanterelle mushrooms go superbly with eggs to make a dish of creamy yellow colours. Lightly boiled potatoes or wholewheat bread and butter are better accompaniments than toast.

125–225g (4–8oz) chanterelle mushrooms (depending on how many you can find)
50g (2oz) butter
8 eggs
freshly ground black pepper

Thinly slice the chanterelles. Melt the butter in a heavy saucepan on a low heat. Mix in the chanterelles and cook them for 10 minutes, stirring occasionally.

While they are cooking, beat the eggs with the pepper. Stir them into the mushrooms and keep stirring on a low heat until they are set to a creamy scramble. Serves 4.

CHANTERELLE

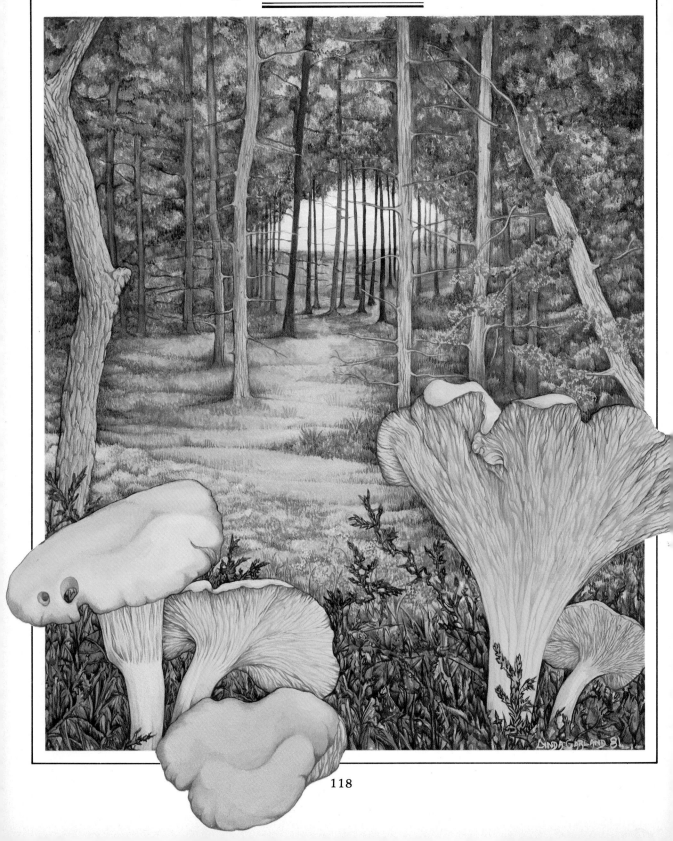

FENNEL

Availability

Fennel came originally from the shores of the Mediterranean but it now grows wild in most of the temperate areas of Europe, particularly in France and Germany. In Britain, it can be found round the coast of Wales and the south west and south of England. It is a cultivated garden herb in the United States but some escapes can be found. In Australia it has also escaped into the wild, particularly along railway lines.

Fennel grows best on dry limestone soil near the coast. It can be found on sea cliffs and along shoreline walks. It will occasionally grow on chalky soil further inland where it favours sunny banks and railway embankments and stony, rubbly ground.

The feathery leaves of fennel appear in spring (March to April in the northern hemisphere and September to October in Australasia) and can be picked until autumn. The plants grow increasingly taller until the yellow flowers appear in late summer (July to August in the northern hemisphere/January to February in Australasia).

The leaves are best used fresh and should be cut from the plant with scissors. Use them as soon as possible after picking as they will quickly become limp.

To collect the seeds, cut off the whole heads when they have finished flowering and hang them up in the dark in paper bags. To dry the stalks, cut off the leaves and flower heads. Hang the stalks up in bunches. When they are dry, break them into lengths of about 10–15 cm (4–6 inches) and store them in airtight jars.

To use the stalks as a flavouring for grilled or broiled food

Heat the grill/broiler to the highest temperature, getting the rack very hot. Cover the hot rack with dried fennel stalks and return them to the grill/broiler so they begin to char. Lay meat or fish on top of the stalks and grill/broil them to your liking.

Pork and lamb chops, steaks, liver and kidneys can all be given this treatment. So, too, can oily fish such as mackerel and herring.

For fish, whether whole or filleted, cover the rack with foil if it is one of the open wire kinds. Turn whole fish once during cooking. Fish fillets should be grilled/broiled on the cut side only and will cook through beautifully provided the rack and stalks are very hot. Put one piece of stalk on top of each fillet during the cooking, or scatter the fillets with fennel seeds or chopped fresh fennel.

Fennel stalks can also be placed over a barbecue before placing the meat on the rack. They will give a delicious, aromatic smoking flavour.

Coddled Potatoes with Fennel Seed

These potatoes are not quite mashed and not quite whole. They have a light, creamy texture and are very tasty.

675 g (1½ lbs) boiling potatoes
25 g (1 oz) butter
5 ml (1 teaspoon) dried fennel seed

Boil the potatoes in their skins until they are just tender. Drain them and let them steam dry. Skin them and cut them into 2.5 cm (1 inch) dice.

Melt the butter in a saucepan on a low heat and scatter in the fennel seed. Fold in the potatoes. Cover them and leave them on the heat for 5 minutes so the bottom layer just begins to brown. Stir them, mixing in the brown pieces. Serves 4.

Cauliflower with Fennel

Serve this cauliflower with white fish, lamb or chicken.

1 medium sized cauliflower
30 ml (2 tablespoons) chopped fennel
150 ml (¼ pint) stock
15 ml (1 tablespoon) tomato purée
15 ml (1 tablespoon) olive oil

Break the cauliflower into small fleurettes and keep the best inner leaves.

Put the stock, tomato purée and oil into a saucepan and bring them to the boil. Turn the cauliflower in the mixture, getting it well coated. Put in the fennel. Cover the pan and set it on a moderate heat for 12 minutes, turning the cauliflower once.

By the end of the cooking time, most of the stock should have evaporated and the cauliflower will be slightly pink and flecked with fennel. Serves 4.

FENNEL

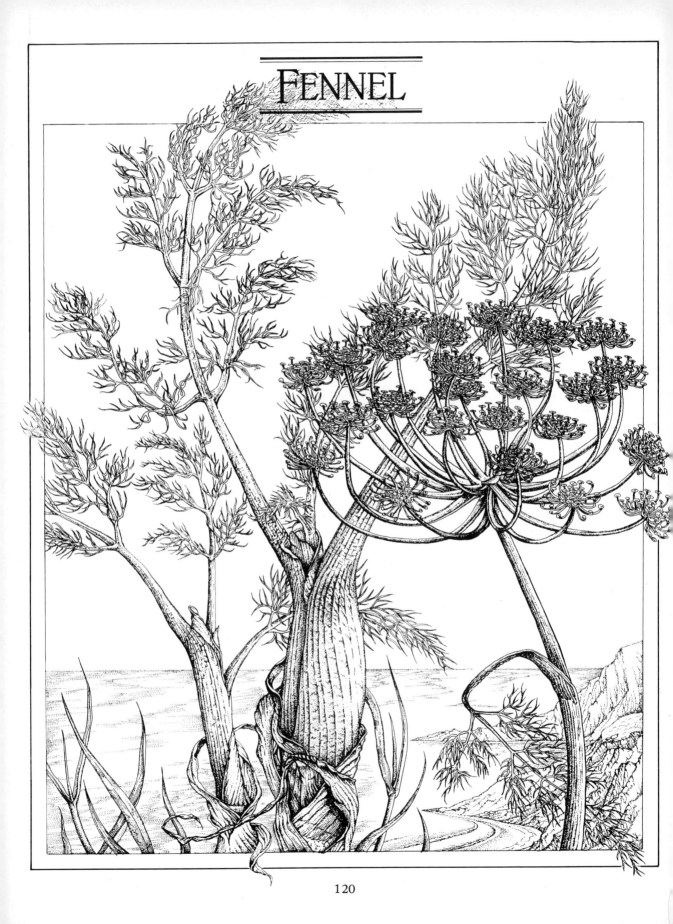

Mackerel Grilled/Broiled with Fennel Stalks

Fennel is said to make oily fish more digestible. Here is another way of grilling mackerel with fennel stalks which can be either fresh or dried. The seeds are used for a savoury butter.

4 small mackerel
juice 1 lemon
Freshly ground black pepper
24 thin pieces fennel stalk 2.5 cm (1 inch) long, bruised
4 thick pieces fennel stalk 7.5 cm–10 cm (3–4 inches) long
fennel seed butter:
125 g (4 oz) butter
grated rind and juice ½ lemon
10 ml (2 teaspoons) fennel seeds

Clean the mackerel, cut off the fins but leave the heads. Van Dyke (cut a V in their tails). Cut three diagonal slits in both sides of each mackerel, running backwards and downwards from head to tail and through almost to the backbone.

Brush the mackerel inside and outside and in the slits with lemon juice. Season them very well with the pepper. Push a short piece of fennel stalk into each slit and put one large one inside the belly. Leave the mackerel to stand for four hours at room temperature.

Meanwhile, cream the butter and beat in the lemon rind and as much juice, drop by drop, as the butter will take. Beat in the fennel seeds. Form the butter into a roll, wrap it in waxed paper and chill to make it firm.

When you are ready to cook, preheat the grill/broiler to the highest temperature and if you have an open wire rack cover it with foil. Lay the mackerel on the hot rack and grill/broil them for 4–5 minutes on each side so they are cooked through and beginning to brown.

Cut the butter into round pats and serve it separately, to put on the mackerel. Serves 4.

Sprats (or very small Herrings) steamed with Fennel and Lemon

This way of cooking sprats (or very small herrings) seals in all the natural flavours.

675 g (1½ lbs) sprats (or very small herrings)
30 ml (2 tablespoons) chopped fennel
1 lemon

Head and gut the fish. Lay them on a large piece of foil in no more than two layers and sprinkle them with the fennel. Cut the peel and pith from the lemon and finely chop the flesh. Scatter the pieces over the fish. Seal the edges of the foil together.

Lay the parcel in the top of a large steamer or in a large collander. Set it over boiling water and cover it with the steamer or saucepan lid. Steam the fish for 20 minutes.

Unwrap them carefully so as to retain the juices. Serve them with the juices and the pieces of lemon spooned over them. Serves 4.

Medicinal

A face pack to smooth wrinkles

90 ml (6 tablespoons) chopped fennel
1 egg white
juice 1 lemon
50 g (2 oz) powdered clay (fuller's earth)

Put the fennel, egg white and lemon juice into a bowl and gradually mix in the powdered clay (fuller's earth) so you have a still paste. Wash your face with warm water and dry it. Spread the paste over your face and lie still, trying not to laugh, for 15 minutes. Gently sponge off the pack with warm water and pat your face dry.

To brighten tired eyes: Infuse 5 ml (1 teaspoon) chopped fennel leaves in 250 ml (8 fl oz) boiling water until the liquid is cool. Strain and use the infusion to bathe your eyes.

To ease sore eyes and eyelids: Make a decoction by boiling 50 g (2 oz) fennel seeds in 1 litre (1¾ pints) water for 5 minutes. Strain the decoction into a jug. Put your head over the jug and cover it with a towel. Blink your eyes over the steam.

Fennel compress for inflamed eyelids: Crush 15 ml (1 tablespoon) fennel seeds and infuse them in 500 ml (16 fl oz) boiling water for 15 minutes. Strain. When the infusion is lukewarm, dip pads of cotton wool into it and place them over the eyes for 15 minutes.

For headaches and migraines: Make up the decoction as for the fennel compress. Use it, lukewarm, for bathing the forehead and temples three times a day.

An appetite stimulant: Macerate 50 g (2 oz) fennel seeds in 1 litre (1¾ pints) red or white wine for 10 days. Strain the wine. Drink 1 wineglassful after the midday and evening meals.

For flatulence: Infuse 5 ml (1 teaspoon) crushed fennel seeds in 250 ml (8 fl oz) boiling water for 10 minutes. Strain and drink the whole amount twice a day.
Or, simmer 5 ml (1 teaspoon) seeds in 250 ml (8 fl oz) milk for 10 minutes. Drink it as hot as possible.

For indigestion and hiccoughs in small children: Infuse 5 ml (1 teaspoon) crushed seeds in 250 ml (8 fl oz) boiling water for 15 minutes. Drink the whole amount, warm, 2–3 times a day. Sweeten with honey if required.

Veterinary

For all gastric ailments in animals, including colic and acute constipation, feed two handfuls of the raw herb twice a day. For indigestion in animals, make an infusion of the seeds and add it to the drinking water.

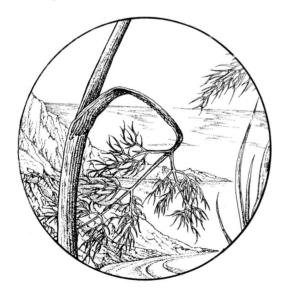

FIELD POPPY

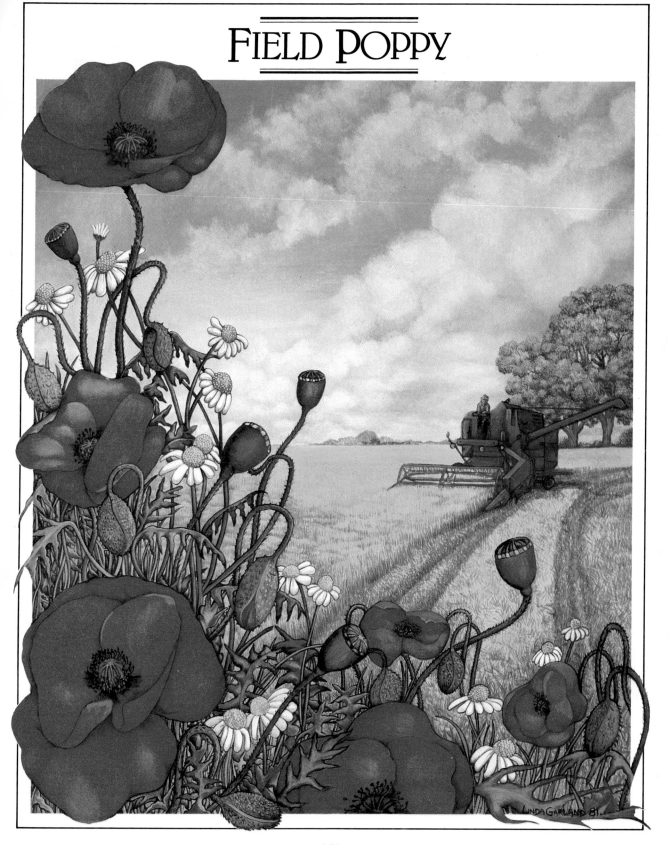

PAPAVER RHOEAS

Local Names: Blind Eyes, Butterfly Ladies, Canker-Rose,
Cheese Bowls, Cock's Comb, Corn Poppy, Corn Rose,
Earaches, Fireflout, Lightnings, Old Woman's Petticoat,
Pepper Boxes, Poppet, Redcap, Red Rags, Red Soldiers,
Sleepyhead, Thunderbolt, Thunderflower, Wart Flower.

Availability

The field poppy grows throughout Europe, mainly in the more southern regions. It is widespread in Britain, although less common in Wales, northern Scotland and northwest England. It can only occasionally be found in the United States but here the many coloured Shirley Poppy, which is frequently cultivated, can be used in the same ways. Field poppies are not common to Australia, but there are many cultivated varieties. Dried poppy seed is available.

Field poppies grow along the edges of cornfields and arable land, by the sides of roads, in gardens and on waste ground. Where land has been recently disturbed they can sometimes spring up in their thousands, creating a spectacular, blazing display of red.

Poppies flower from mid-summer until autumn (June to October in the northern hemisphere/December to April in Australasia). Gather the petals when they are in full flower and either use them right away or dry them on racks. The leaves are best picked when the flower is still in bud. If you wish to gather the seed heads for medicinal purposes, cut them as soon as the petals drop off.

To collect the seeds, wait until the seed heads are beginning to turn a grey-brown colour and small holes appear just underneath the flat tops. Cut them with about 15 cm (6 inches) of stalk still attached. Put them, head down, into paper bags and hang them up for about four days. Give the bag a shake and the seeds will drop out into the bottom. Store the seeds in air and light-tight jars. They will be smaller than the poppy seeds that you can buy but will still have the same nutty flavour.

A Poppy Seed Topping for Bread

Poppies and corn not only look superb together in the field. When the corn is ground and the seeds collected, the flavour of each enhances the other.

Make wholewheat bread and shape your loaves in the usual way, either on baking sheets or in bread tins. Brush the loaves with beaten egg and scatter them quite thickly with poppy seeds. Slash the tops with several diagonal cuts and then leave the loaves to prove.

Bake the loaves for the required amount of time and they will have a glossy, deep brown top, speckled with poppy seeds.

Poppy Bread

When making plain bread dough set aside a 225 g (8 oz) portion to make poppy bread. It makes a lovely soft loaf with a nutty flavour.

plain bread dough made with 225 g (8 oz) wholewheat flour
25 g (1 oz) butter, softened
30 ml (2 tablespoons) plus 5 ml (1 teaspoon) poppy seeds
1 egg, beaten

Heat the oven to Reg 6/200C/400F. Knead the dough lightly and then knead in the butter and the 30 ml (2 tablespoons) poppy seeds. Form the dough lightly and then knead in the butter and the sheet. Brush it with beaten egg and scatter with the remaining poppy seeds. Make a small cross cut in the top.

Cover the loaf with a clean towel and leave it in a warm place to prove for 15 minutes. Bake it for 40 minutes and put it on a wire rack to cool.

Honey and Poppy Seed Cake

Poppy seeds in cakes go particularly well with honey.

175 g (6 oz) butter, softened
225 g (8 oz) honey
225 g (8 oz) wholewheat flour
5 ml (1 teaspoon) baking powder
5 ml (1 teaspoon) ground cinnamon
2 eggs, beaten
30 ml (2 tablespoons) poppy seeds
50 g (2 oz) walnuts, chopped
butter for greasing a 900 g (2 lb) loaf tin

Heat the oven to Reg 4/180C/350F. Beat the butter to a cream. Beat in the honey.

Toss the flour with the baking powder and cinnamon. Add it to the butter, alternately with the eggs. Fold in the poppy seeds and walnuts.

Put the mixture into the prepared tin and smooth the top. Bake the cake for 40 minutes, or until a skewer inserted into the centre comes out clean.

Cool the cake in the tin for 5 minutes and turn it onto a wire rack to cool completely.

Poppy Seed Cookies

These cookies are light and crisp, with a nutty flavour.

175 g (6 oz) wholewheat flour
2.5 ml (½ teaspoon) bicarbonate of soda
2.5 ml (½ teaspoon) ground cinnamon
75 g (3 oz) butter, softened
175 g (6 oz) light brown (Barbados) sugar
1 egg, beaten
45 ml (3 tablespoons) poppy seeds

Heat the oven to Reg 5/190C/375F. Butter and flour some baking sheets. Toss the flour with the baking soda and cinnamon.

Cream the butter in a bowl and beat in the sugar. Beat in the egg, a little at a time and then stir in the flour and poppy seeds.

Drop 7.5 ml (1½ teaspoon) amounts onto the baking sheets, 5 cm (2 inches) apart. Flatten the portions slightly with a wet fork.

Bake them for 10 minutes or until they are golden brown. As they will still be very soft, cool them for 5 minutes on the baking sheets and then carefully lift them onto wire racks, using a spatula. Let them cool completely. Makes about 40.

Chicken with Fennel and Poppy Seeds

If no fennel is available for this recipe, parsley can be used instead.

60 ml (4 tablespoons) olive oil
juice 1 lemon
1 clove garlic, crushed with a pinch sea salt
freshly ground black pepper
60 ml (4 tablespoons) chopped fennel
125 g (4 oz) breadcrumbs
30 ml (2 tablespoons) poppy seeds

Cut the chicken into 8 pieces. In a bowl, mix together the oil, lemon juice, garlic, pepper and fennel. Turn the chicken pieces in the mixture and leave them to marinate for four hours at room temperature.

Heat the oven to Reg 6/200C/400F. Put the chicken pieces, skin side up, in a large, flat dish and put them into the oven for 25 minutes.

While they are cooking, mix the breadcrumbs and poppy seeds into the remaining marinade. Spoon this mixture over the chicken and put the dish back into the oven for a further 20 minutes, so the breadcrumbs brown and the surface becomes crisp. Serves 4.

Pineapple, Poppy Seed and Walnut Salad

Serve this salad as a first course.

1 small pineapple
275 ml (½ pint) natural yoghurt
10 ml (2 teaspoons) ground coriander
1 clove garlic, crushed with a pinch sea salt
freshly ground black pepper
30 ml (2 tablespoons) poppy seeds
50 g (2 oz) chopped walnuts

Cut the rind and husk from the pineapple and cut the flesh into 8 slices. Core them and cut them in half.

Arrange the halves in an overlapping line on each of four small plates. Beat the yoghurt with the coriander, garlic and pepper and spoon it over the pineapple. Scatter the poppy seeds in a line down the centre and the walnuts over the top.

Mixed Salad with Poppy Seeds

Poppy seeds can add a nutty richness to side salads, especially if they are left soaking in the dressing for a while before serving.

350 g (12 oz) carrots
6 large celery sticks
1 green pepper
1 large, crisp eating apple
30 ml (2 tablespoons) poppy seeds
60 ml (4 tablespoons) sesame or walnut oil
30 ml (2 tablespoons) cider vinegar
1 clove garlic, crushed with a pinch sea salt
freshly ground black pepper
little freshly grated nutmeg

Coarsely grate the carrots. Finely chop the celery. Core, deseed and chop the pepper. Core and chop the apple. Mix them all in a salad bowl with the poppy seeds.

Beat the remaining ingredients together and fold them into the salad. Let the salad stand for 15 minutes before serving. Serves 4.

Medicinal

A general tonic: Eat 10 ml (2 teaspoons) poppy seeds every morning, either with a spoon or sprinkled on breakfast cereal or fruit.

For insomnia: Infuse five whole flower heads or green seed capsules in 250 ml (8 fl oz) boiling water for 10 minutes. Strain and sweeten with honey. Drink the whole amount, hot, on going to bed.

For general exciteability: Drink the above infusion several times during the day.

For tonsilitis: Infuse 45 ml (3 tablespoons) dried poppy petals in 1 litre (1¾ pints) boiling water for 10 minutes. Strain and sweeten with honey. Drink four cups of the infusion throughout the day.

For bronchitis: Drink one cup of the above infusion one hour after each of the three main meals.

Veterinary

Poppy seeds, mixed with olive oil and honey, are given by the Arabs to fretful horses.
One handful of poppy seeds is a daily tonic for all animals.
In cases of pneumonia, pleurisy and asthma in animals, feed them two handfuls of the whole plant (except the roots) twice a day.

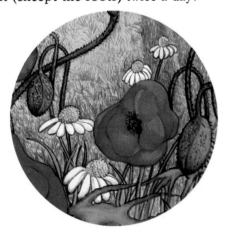

TANSY

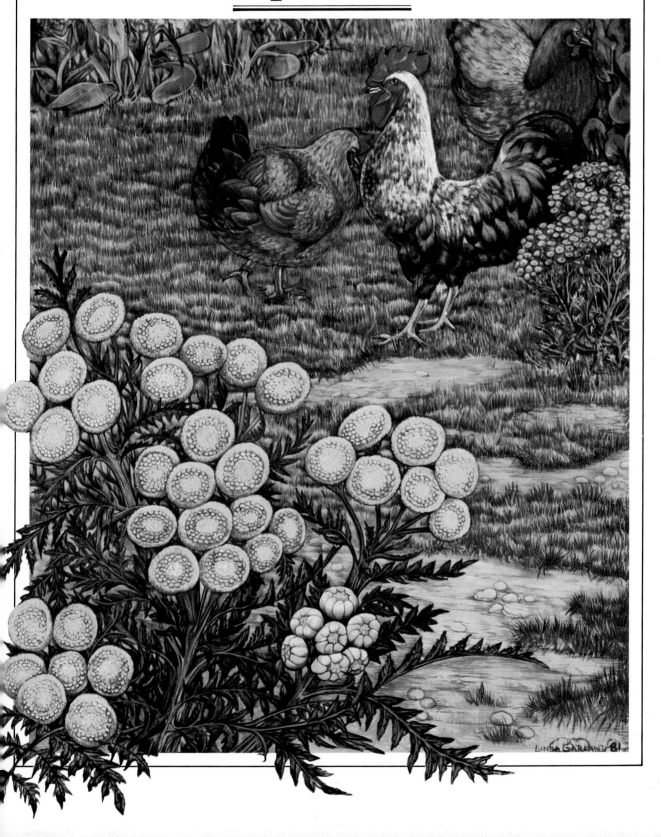

Availability

Tansy grows throughout Britain, Europe, Scandinavia and the United States. In Australia it is not a wild plant but can be very easily grown — and is quite common in gardens. It likes damp soil and can be found growing on the edges of woodlands, by roadsides, on damp waste ground and along grassy verges. It also grows along river banks and on sandy or earth sea cliffs.

The leaves of tansy start to grow in spring but are not easily identifiable until the flowers appear in late summer (July in the northern hemisphere/ January in Australasia). Both leaves and flowers can be picked until autumn. Snip them off the main plants with scissors. The youngest leaves growing in the centre of the plant are the softest and best flavoured and as long as the stems are tender they can be chopped and used with the leaf. The stems from larger, older leaves are tough and bitter and should be discarded after you have stripped away the leaves.

For medicinal uses, cut the whole plant just above the ground just as it is coming into flower.

Potato and Tansy Salad

The slightly bitter flavour of tansy goes well with the blander flavour of potatoes.

900 g (2 lbs) small new potatoes
90 ml (6 tablespoons) olive oil
45 ml (3 tablespoons) white wine vinegar
freshly ground black pepper
30 ml (2 tablespoons) chopped tansy
60 ml (4 tablespoons) chopped chives
petals from 6 marigold heads

Boil the potatoes in their skins, While they are cooking, beat together the olive oil, vinegar and pepper.

Drain the potatoes, skin them if wished and cut them into thick slices. Put them into a bowl. Fold in the dressing, tansy and chives. Scatter the marigold petals over the top.

Serve the salad while it is still warm. Serves 4.

Tansy and Corn Au Gratin

If this is made in small dishes it can be served as a first course. Made in one large dish, it can be served as a lunch or supper dish or as a substantial side vegetable.

4 corn cobs
1 large onion
25 g (1 oz) butter
30 ml (2 tablespoons) wholewheat flour
275 ml (½ pint) milk
pinch cayenne pepper
30 ml (2 tablespoons) chopped tansy
175 g (6 oz) Cheddar cheese, grated

Cut the corn from the cobs and finely chop the onion. Melt the butter in a saucepan on a low heat. Stir in the onion and corn. Cover them and cook them gently for 10 minutes.

Stir in the flour and cook it for ½ minute. Pour in the milk and bring it to the boil, stirring. Add the cayenne pepper and tansy. Simmer everything for 2 minutes, stirring frequently, so the sauce becomes very thick. Take the pan from the heat and beat in two thirds of the cheese.

Either divide the mixture between four individual soufflé dishes or pour it all into one ovenproof dish. Scatter the remaining cheese on top. Put the dishes under a preheated high grill/broiler for the cheese to melt and just begin to brown. Serves 4.

Tansy and Bacon Omelette

Like sage, another bitter herb, tansy goes well with bacon.

50 g (2 oz) smoked bacon
15 g (½ oz) butter
¼ medium onion, thinly sliced
2 eggs
15 ml (1 tablespoon) water
10 ml (2 teaspoons) chopped tansy
freshly ground black pepper

Finely chop the bacon. Melt the butter in an omelette pan on a low heat. Put in the bacon and onion and cook them until they begin to brown.

Beat the eggs with the water, tansy and pepper. Pour them into the pan and stir them around with a fork. Cook the omelette until the underside is brown and the top set. Roll it up and slide it onto a warm plate. Serves 1.

To make more omelettes, first cook all the bacon and onion together. Take out all but the amount that you need for one omelette. Beat the two eggs separately for each one. Keep the first omelette warm and add bacon and onion to the pan to make one more omelette. You may also need a little more butter.

Tansy Meat Loaf

Hot or cold, this meat loaf makes a tasty main meal. Thin slices are also very good in sandwiches.

675 g (1½ lbs) good quality sausage meat (not too highly seasoned)
8 black peppercorns
3 allspice berries
pinch sea salt
30 ml (2 tablespoons) chopped tansy

Heat the oven to Reg 5/190 C/375 F. Put the sausagemeat into a bowl. Crush the peppercorns, allspice berries and salt together and add them to the sausagemeat. Add the tansy and mix well. Press the mixture into a 450 g (1 lb) loaf tin and bake it for 50 minutes.

To serve the loaf hot, cut it into slices while it is still in the tin. To serve it cold, let it cool completely in the tin and then turn it out. Serves 4.

Pork Chops with Tansy Mustard

4 loin pork chops
30 ml (2 tablespoons) chopped tansy
30 ml (2 tablespoons) dried mustard powder
5 ml (1 teaspoon) honey
60 ml (4 tablespoons) dry cider

Cut the rind from the chops. Heat the grill/broiler to the highest temperature. Mix together the tansy, mustard, honey and cider.

Lay the chops on the hot grill/broiler and spread them with half the mustard mixture. Grill/broil them until the mustard side is a good brown. Turn them over, spread them with the remaining mustard mixture and brown the second side. Serves 4.

Tansy Simmer Pot

Tansy is a good herb to use in beef stews and casseroles of mince-meat, like this all-in-one main meal.

450 g (1 lb) string beans
2 yellow squashes, or 450 g (1 lb) courgettes (zucchini)
175 g (6 oz) carrots
25 g (1 oz) butter
1 large onion, finely chopped
1 clove garlic, finely chopped
1.5 ml (¼ teaspoon) cayenne pepper
450 g (1 lb) minced or ground beef
30 ml (2 tablespoons) chopped tansy
45 ml (3 tablespoons) chopped parsley
150 ml (¼ pint) dry red wine

String and slice the beans. Deseed the squashes, peel them if necessary and chop them. (Or, wipe and chop the courgettes (zucchini)). Finely chop the carrots.

Melt the butter in a large saucepan or flameproof casserole on a low heat. Mix in the onion and garlic and soften them. Stir in the cayenne pepper.

Raise the heat. Add the beef and break it up well. Stir it around until it browns. Mix in the tansy and parsley, beans and squash. Pour in the wine and bring it to the boil. Cover and simmer for 35 minutes. Serves 4.

To keep flies away: Hang a bunch of tansy in the kitchen. Meat can also be rubbed with tansy to keep off the flies.

Medicinal

For sprains and rheumatic pains: Boil 50 g (2 oz) tansy leaves and flowers in 1.15 litres (2 pints) water for 15 minutes. Strain. Dip a soft cloth in the hot decoction and lay it on the aching part. Hold the cloth in place with a bandage and change it every four hours.

For hysteria and rheumatic pains: Boil 50 g (1 oz) tansy leaves and flowers in 575 ml (1 pint) boiling water for 15 minutes. Strain, sweeten with honey and take in frequent wineglassful doses.

A digestive tonic useful in cases of dyspepsia and anaemia: Infuse 15 ml (1 tablespoon) chopped tansy leaves in 250 ml (8 fl oz) boiling water for 10 minutes. Strain and drink the whole amount before each of the two main meals.

Or, macerate 50 g (2 oz) chopped tansy leaves in 1 litre (1¾ pints) wine for 8 days. Strain and bottle. Drink one wine glass full after each of the two main meals.

To ease cramp: Infuse 60 ml (4 tablespoons) chopped tansy leaves in 575 ml (1 pint) boiling water for 10 minutes. Strain. Drink one cupful.

For indigestion: Infuse 60 ml (4 tablespoons) chopped tansy leaves in 500 ml (16 fl oz) boiling water for 10 minutes. Strain and sweeten with honey. Drink the infusion in two halves, one hour apart.

During pregnancy: For morning sickness, failing appetite, nausea, threatened abortion, put 15 ml (1 tablespoon) chopped tansy leaves into a saucepan with 750 ml (1½ pints) water and bring them to simmering point. Cover and keep just under boiling for 3 minutes. Remove from the heat and let stand 3 hours. Strain. Drink 15 ml (1 tablespoon) three times a day before meals.

Veterinary

Cows and sheep will eat tansy but goats and pigs refuse to touch it.

The seeds of tansy are a worm expellant. Feed the animal 50 g (2 oz) daily.

For general debility, feed one handful of the leaves and flowers twice a day.

To prevent abortion, make a decoction by boiling a handful of the leaves and flowers in 1.15 litres (2 pints) water for 15 minutes. Add honey and make the animal drink 275 ml (½ pint) twice a day.

To ease sprains, put tansy leaves and flowers in a muslin bag and put them into boiling water for 15 minutes. Put the bag, while still warm, on the aching limb.

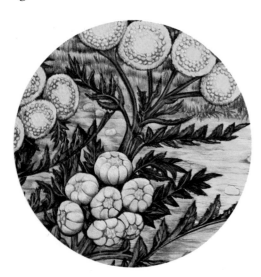

Yarrow

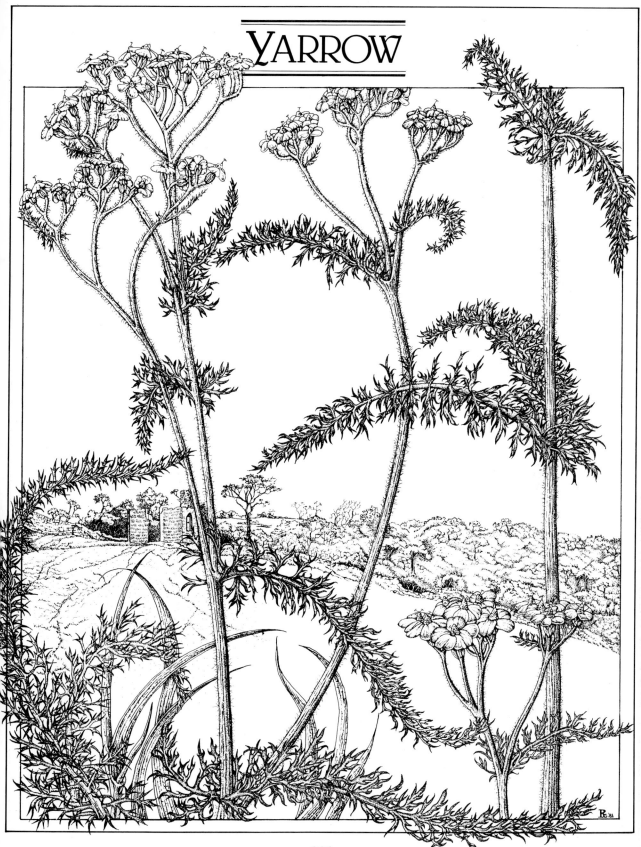

ACHILLEA MILLEFOLIUM
Local Names: Angel Flower, Baldwort, Bloodwort,
Bunch o' Daisies, Cammock, Carpenter's Weed,
Devil's Plaything, Goose Tongue, Green Arrow,
Hemming-and-Sewing, Hundred Leaved Grass,
Melancholy, Mother of Thousands, Milfoil, Nosebleed,
Old Man's Pepper, Sanguinary, Sneezewort, Soldier's
Woundwort, Staunchwort, Sweet Nuts, Thousand Leaf
Clover/Grass, Traveller's Ease, Wild Pepper, Yallow,
Yarra-Grass, Yarrel, Yarroway.

Availability

Yarrow grows throughout Britain, Scandinavia, Europe and all over the United States except for the extreme south. In Australia, it is mainly found in cultivation where it quickly becomes a weed.

It grows best in grassy places, in meadows and pastures, by roadsides and country lanes and in gardens. It can also be found on sunny, grassy banks and on the lower slopes of hills.

Yarrow flowers in late summer (July to August in the northern hemisphere/January to February in Australasia) and is best when the flowers are just opening. For cooking, either cut or break the leaves from the stems and use them immediately or cut the whole plants and keep them in a jar of water, taking off the leaves as you need them. They will keep fresh for up to three days.

For drying and using medicinally, cut and hang up the whole plants. When they are dry, crumble the leaves and flowers and store them in light and airtight containers.

Curried Yarrow Soup

Cooked yarrow has a spicy spinach-like flavour that goes exceptionally well with curry.

40 g (1½ oz) butter
2 medium onions, finely chopped
1 clove garlic, finely chopped
10 ml (2 teaspoons) curry powder
5 ml (1 teaspoon) ground turmeric
30 ml (2 tablespoons) wholewheat flour
850 ml (1½ pints) stock
125 g (4 oz) yarrow leaves, finely chopped
275 ml (½ pint) natural yoghurt

Melt the butter in a saucepan on a low heat. Stir in the onions, garlic, curry powder and turmeric and cook them until the onions are soft.

Stir in the flour and cook for 1 minute. Stir in the stock and bring it to the boil. Add the yarrow and simmer the soup, uncovered, for 15 minutes.

Take the pan from the heat, stir in the yoghurt and serve. Serves 4.

Beetroot (Beet) and Yarrow Salad

In salads, yarrow has a fresh, slightly bitter taste, so it complements ingredients that have a slightly sweet flavour, such as beetroot.

450 g (1 lb) small beetroot (beet)
45 ml (3 tablespoons) chopped yarrow
60 ml (4 tablespoons) soured cream
15 ml (1 tablespoon) red wine vinegar

Boil the beetroot or beet until they are tender. Peel and dice them and put them into a bowl with the yarrow.

Mix together the soured cream and vinegar and fold them into the beetroot. Serves 4.

Butter (Lima) Beans in Soured Cream Sauce

These butter beans can be served as a side dish, or with pasta as a main course.

225 g (8 oz) butter (lima) beans
60 ml (4 tablespoons) chopped yarrow
1 large onion, thinly sliced
150 ml (¼ pint) soured cream

Soak the butter beans and boil them until they are tender. Drain them and reserve the cooking liquid.

Put 150 ml (¼ pint) of the cooking liquid into a saucepan, and bring it to the boil. Put in the yarrow and onion and boil gently until the onion is tender and the liquid is almost completely reduced (about 15 minutes). Stir in the soured cream. Fold in the beans and heat them through. Serves 4.

Yarrow Kedgeree

The fresh, spiciness of yarrow goes well in a curried kedgeree.

225 g (8 oz) long grain brown rice
675 g (1½ lbs) smoked cod
1 bayleaf
1 blade mace
5 ml (1 teaspoon) black peppercorns
40 g (1 oz) butter
1 large onion, thinly sliced
10 ml (2 teaspoons) curry powder
10 ml (2 teaspoons) ground turmeric
50 g (2 oz) sultanas
60 ml (4 tablespoons) chopped yarrow

Cook the rice in lightly salted water until it is tender. Drain it, run cold water through it and drain it again.

Put the cod into a shallow pan with the bayleaf,

mace and peppercorns. Cover it and bring it slowly to the boil. Simmer it for 10 minutes. Lift it out of the pan, flake it and remove any bones.

Melt the butter in a frying pan on a low heat. Stir in the onion, curry powder and turmeric and cook them until the onion is soft. Mix in the rice, sultanas, fish and yarrow and fork them around until they have all heated through. Serve as soon as possible. Serves 4.

Chicken with Yarrow stuffing

one 1.575 kg (3½ lb) roasting chicken
25 g (1 oz) butter, softened
5 ml (1 teaspoon) ground ginger
1.5 ml (¼ teaspoon) cayenne pepper
stuffing:
15 g (½ oz) butter
1 medium onion, finely chopped
1 clove garlic, finely chopped
5 ml (1 teaspoon) ground ginger
1.5 ml (¼ teaspoon) cayenne pepper
75 g (3 oz) fresh breadcrumbs
60 ml (4 tablespoons) chopped yarrow
juice ½ lemon

Heat the oven to Reg 6/200 C/400 F. Cream the softened butter with the ginger, cayenne and pepper.

To make the stuffing, melt the butter in a frying pan on a low heat. Mix in the onion, garlic, ginger and cayenne and cook them until the onion is soft. Take the pan from the heat and mix in the breadcrumbs, yarrow and lemon juice.

Fill the chicken with the stuffing and truss it. Put it on a rack in a roasting tin and spread it with the spiced butter. Cover it completely with foil and roast it for 1 hour. Remove the foil and cook for a further 30 minutes so the skin browns well. Serves 4.

For severe colds and influenza: Infuse 15 ml (1 tablespoon) each dried yarrow and peppermint in 275 ml (½ pint) boiling water for 10 minutes. Strain, sweeten with honey and add a pinch of cayenne pepper. Drink the whole amount, fasting, four times a day.

For indigestion: Infuse 10 ml (2 teaspoons) chopped fresh flowers in 250 ml (8 fl oz) boiling water for 10 minutes. Strain. Drink the whole amount twice a day between meals.

For poor circulation, varicose veins, menstrual disturbances: Bring 50 g (2 oz) dried yarrow to the boil in 1 litre (1¾ pints) water. Take it from the heat and leave it to stand for 10 minutes. Drink 2–3 cups a day.

To dry oily hair: Rinse the hair with the above decoction after washing. Also, drink an infusion of yarrow twice a day, 10 ml (2 teaspoons) to 250 ml (8 fl oz) boiling water.

Veterinary

Sheep and goats grazing on dry ground will seek out yarrow as a tonic.

For fevers, pneumonia and colic, put 2 handfuls of the whole herb into 850 ml (1½ pints) water, bring them to just under boiling and keep them there for 3 minutes. Remove the brew from the heat and let it steep for 6 hours. Give 250 ml (8 fl oz) night and morning, fasting.

For wounds, skin eruptions and abscesses, bathe with a stronger brew made in the same way as above but with three handfuls of yarrow to 850 ml (1½ pints) water.

Medicinal

To combat pimples and scabbing, oily skin and open pores and to generally improve the complexion: Boil 50 g (2 oz) dried yarrow in 1 litre (1¾ pints) water for 3 minutes, then let the decoction stand for 10 minutes. Strain it. Rinse the face with it several times a day and let it dry naturally.

For cuts and scrapes: Bathe them with the above decoction.

COMMON PUFFBALL

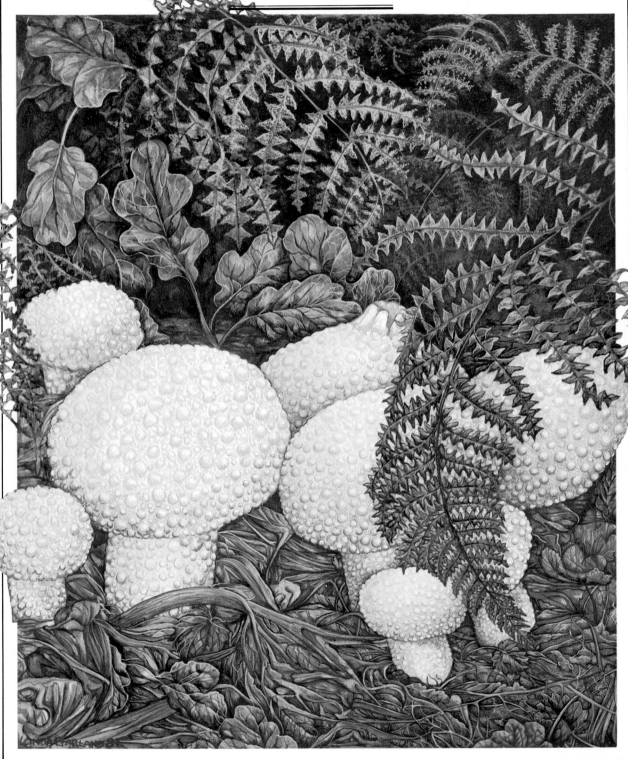

COMMON PUFFBALL
GIANT PUFFBALL

LYCOPERDON PERLATUM
LYCOPERDON GIGANTEUM
Local Names: Common; Devil's Tobacco Pouch
Local Names: Giant; None available

Availability

The common puffball is the more abundant of the two and it grows throughout Britain, Scandinavia, Europe and the United States. In Australia Lycoperdon glabrescens and Lycoperdon pratense are the two varieties found. The first is not usually eaten the second is edible when young and is fairly common.

It can be found in pastures and meadows, on grassy heaths and on lawns. It can occasionally be found in woods under conifer trees. It appears from mid-summer until autumn (June to November in the northern hemisphere) and in Australia from December to January and April to July.

Always pick common puffballs when they are still white or pale cream and small—about 3.5–5 cm (1½–2 inches) across.

Cook them as soon as you can after picking as they carry on maturing in the cupboard and what might have looked to be good specimens one day can be old, dusty ones when you come to cooking them the next.

The giant puffball is one of the most spectacular of fungi, since it can grow to 28 cm (12 inches) across and can be found in meadows and pastures, especially under hedges, during late summer and early autumn.

In the United States there is a related species, Calvatia gigantea, which can be used in the same ways. It can be found from July to September and grows in damp areas, by small streams and drainage ditches and along the edges of meadows. It can be found mostly in the central and eastern states.

When picking a giant puffball, hold it with both hands and very gently twist it from the ground. It should be white. If it is starting to yellow it is past its best.

If you are unable to use all the puffball at once, put it into a plastic bag and put it into the refrigerator. It will stay fresh for up to two days.

Cooking Common Puffballs

If common puffballs are very young, they will not need peeling. If, when you slice them, the skin looks rather tough, it is worthwhile removing it. Peel it away like that on a cultivated mushroom. Common puffballs have a soft, melting texture.

To cook them thinly sliced you need 40 g (1½ oz) butter to 225 g (8 oz) puffballs. Cook them on a medium heat, stirring frequently, for about 3 minutes. Season them with pepper and add a squeeze of lemon juice.

Deep Fried Puffballs with Lemon Butter

Serve this as a first course.

8 common puffballs
2 eggs, beaten
25 g (1 oz) wholewheat flour, seasoned
Deep fat for frying
50 g (2 oz) butter
juice 1½ lemons
60 ml (4 tablespoons) chopped parsley

Cut the puffballs in half lengthways. Dip them into the beaten eggs and then coat with flour. Deep fry them in hot oil until they are brown (about 3 minutes). Drain them on absorbent paper towels. Divide them between four small, individual plates.

Melt the butter in a frying pan on a low heat. Swirl in the lemon juice and parsley. Pour the butter over the mushrooms just before serving. Serves 4.

Cooking a Giant Puffball

Cut the puffball into slices about 1.5 cm (½ inch) thick. If you fry them plainly in butter, keep them on a high heat and brown them quickly on both sides. A low heat gives them a rather sloppy texture.

Before cooking you can dip the slices first in beaten egg and then in seasoned wholewheat flour. Again, fry them quickly. With wholewheat bread and butter and a salad, one slice fried in this way can make a light meal.

Breadcrumbed Puffball Slices with tomato sauce and Cheese

With a rich tomato sauce and a topping of cheese, thick slices from a giant puffball can make a main meal.

4 slices from a giant puffball, about 10 cm by 15 cm (4 by 6 inches) and 1.5 cm (½ inch) thick
2 eggs, beaten
40 g (1½ oz) browned wholewheat breadcrumbs
50 g (2 oz) butter

tomato sauce:
450 g (1 lb) tomatoes
1 small onion, finely chopped
30 ml (2 tablespoons) malt vinegar
pinch salt
freshly ground black pepper
15 g (½ oz) butter
15 ml (1 tablespoon) wholewheat flour
topping:
175 g (6 oz) Cheddar cheese, grated

First, make the sauce. Roughly chop the tomatoes, without peeling them and put them into a saucepan with the onion, vinegar and seasonings. Cover them and set them on a low heat for 30 minutes so you have a thick pulp. Rub it through a sieve or vegetable mill.

Melt the butter in a saucepan on a low heat, stir in the flour and cook it for 1 minute. Stir in the sieved purée and bring it to the boil, stirring. Simmer it for 2 minutes.

Dip the puffball slices into the beaten eggs and then coat them in breadcrumbs. Melt 25 g (1 oz) butter in a large frying pan on a medium heat. Put in two puffball slices and brown them on both sides (about 2 minutes in each side). Remove them and keep them warm. Put in the remaining butter and cook the other two slices in the same way. Replace the first two. Pour in the sauce and bring it to the boil. Simmer, uncovered, for 2 minutes.

Put the puffball slices into a warm serving dish, spoon the sauce over them and scatter the cheese over the top. Serves 4.

Medicinal

In some areas of Europe, slices of giant puffball were once bound onto wounds to stop bleeding and facilitate healing. They were left in place until the wound had healed.

Veterinary

Dried slices of puffball are very effective burned in the smoker when you are collecting honey.

WILD MARJORAM

OREGANUM VULGARE
Local Names: Joy of the Mountain, Organ, Organy

Availability

Wild marjoram grows throughout Britain, Europe and Scandinavia. It can be found all over the United States but is most common in the north eastern states. In Australia it is available from herb nurseries and will grow easily.

Marjoram will grow in all kinds of soil but it loves dry places so you will find it on dry heaths, chalk cliffs, railway embankments and banks by roadsides. It also grows in dry pastures, along hedge banks and edges of woods and on scrubland.

The flowers appear in late summer and can bloom until autumn (July to September in the northern hemisphere/January to March in Australasia). Cut the whole herb when it is flowering.

Both the leaves and flowers can be used in cooked dishes and salads, but the stems should be discarded as they are too tough. The whole sprigs will keep fresh in water for about three days.

Tomato and Wild Marjoram Soup

675 g (1½ lbs) ripe tomatoes
25 g (1 oz) butter
1 large onion, finely chopped
60 ml (4 tablespoons) chopped wild marjoram
425 ml (¾ pint) stock
1 clove garlic, crushed with a pinch sea salt
150 ml (¼ pint) dry sherry

Scald, skin and finely chop the tomatoes. Melt the butter in a saucepan on a low heat. Add the onion and soften it.

Put in the tomatoes and marjoram, cover and cook them for 10 minutes.

Pour in the stock and bring it to the boil. Add the garlic. Cover and simmer for 10 minutes.

Take the pan from the heat and stir in the sherry. Do not boil the soup any more before serving. Serves 4.

String Beans and Wild Marjoram

Marjoram is an excellent herb for flavouring vegetables. It goes particularly well with string beans.

675 g (1½ lbs) string beans
60 ml (4 tablespoons) olive oil
1 large onion, finely chopped
1 clove garlic, finely chopped
60 ml (4 tablespoons) chopped wild marjoram
90 ml (6 tablespoons) water

String and shred the beans. Heat the oil in a saucepan on a low heat. Mix in the onion and garlic and soften them.

Raise the heat and stir in the beans and marjoram. Add the water and let it boil. Cover the pan and cook the beans on a low heat for 15 minutes. They should still be slightly crisp. Serves 4.

Wild Marjoram Pan Pizza

This is a simply made pizza, flavoured both top and bottom with wild marjoram.

base:
250 g (9 oz) wholewheat flour
pinch sea salt
30 ml (2 tablespoons) chopped wild marjoram
60 ml (4 tablespoons) olive oil
125 ml (4 fl oz) water
for frying: 45 ml (3 tablespoons) olive oil
top:
45 ml (3 tablespoons) olive oil
1 large onion, finely chopped
1 clove garlic, finely chopped
225 g (8 oz) tomatoes, scalded, skinned and chopped
30 ml (2 tablespoons) chopped wild marjoram
125 g (4 oz) Cheddar cheese
4 anchovy fillets
4 black olives

For the base, put the flour, salt and marjoram into a bowl. Make a well in the centre and pour in the oil and water. Mix everything to a dough, turn it onto a floured work top and knead it until it is smooth.

For the top, heat the oil in a frying pan on a low heat. Mix in the onion and garlic and soften them. Mix in the tomatoes and marjoram and cook them gently for 10 minutes so they are reduced to a thick pulp.

Grate the cheese. Cut the anchovy fillets in half lengthways. Halve and stone the olives.

Roll out the dough to a round just larger than the base of a 25 cm (10 inch) frying pan. Heat the oil in the frying pan on a low heat. Put in the round of dough, pressing the edges to make them slightly thicker than the middle. Cook for about 5 minutes so the underside browns. Turn the dough and brown the other side. Take the pan from the heat but leave the pizza base in the pan.

Heat the grill/broiler to the highest temperature. Spread the tomato mixture over the pizza base. Top it with the cheese and make a pattern on the cheese with the anchovies and olives. Put the pan under the grill/broiler so the cheese melts and the anchovies and olives begin to sizzle. Cut the pizza into four and serve it straight from the pan. Serves 4.

Sauté of Beef with Wild Marjoram

900g (2lbs) beef skirt (flank steak)
45ml (3 tablespoons) olive oil
25g (1oz) butter
1 large onion, finely chopped
1 clove garlic, finely chopped
15ml (1 tablespoon) wholewheat flour
150ml (¼ pint) stock
150ml (¼ pint) dry red wine
30ml (2 tablespoons) chopped wild marjoram
grated rind ½ lemon
175g (6oz) mushrooms, thinly sliced

Cut the beef into pieces about 5cm (2 inches) square. Heat the oil and butter in a large frying pan on a high heat. When they stop foaming, put in the pieces of beef and brown them on both sides. Do this in two batches if necessary. Lower the heat. Put in the onion and garlic and soften them. Stir in the flour until it begins to brown. Pour in the stock and wine and bring them to the boil. Add the marjoram, lemon rind and mushrooms and replace the beef. Cover and simmer for 1 hour. Serves 4.

Herbed Pork Patties

These are juicy, herb flavoured patties with a golden, crispy outside.

675g (1½lbs) streaky pork
30ml (2 tablespoons) chopped wild marjoram
4 sage leaves, chopped
12 black peppercorns
4 juniper berries
2.5ml (½ teaspoon) sea salt
2 eggs, beaten
40g (1½oz) wholewheat flour, seasoned

Trim the pork and slice. Lay the slices in a flat dish, overlapping as little as possible. Scatter them with the herbs. Crush together the peppercorns, juniper berries, and salt and sprinkle them over the pork. Leave the pork for 4 hours at room temperature.

Finely mince the pork and form it into 8 round, flat patties. Coat them in flour, dip them in the beaten egg and coat them in flour again. They should be quite dry.

Heat the grill/broiler to the highest temperature and if you have an open, wire rack, cover it with foil. Lay the patties on the hot rack and grill/broil them until they are golden brown on each side. Serve them hot. Apple sauce is a good accompaniment. Serves 4.

Veal Escalopes with Wild Marjoram

Wild marjoram is the perfect herb for meats. It is fragrant but fresher and spicier than the cultivated kinds.

4 veal escalopes
50g (2oz) wholewheat flour, seasoned
25g (1oz) butter
30ml (2 tablespoons) olive oil
1 large onion, finely chopped
1 clove garlic, finely chopped
150ml (¼ pint) dry sherry
90ml (3floz) stock
30ml (2 tablespoons) chopped wild marjoram

Coat the veal in the flour. Put them on a firm surface and bat them flat with a rolling pin. Heat the butter and oil together in a large frying pan on a high heat. When the foam subsides, put in the veal pieces and brown them on both sides. Remove them.

Lower the heat, put in the onion and garlic and soften them. Pour in the sherry and stock and bring them to the boil. Add the wild marjoram. Put the veal back into the pan. Cover them and simmer them for 20 minutes.

Serve the veal with the small amount of sauce that is left spooned over them. Serves 4.

Medicinal

For a stiff neck, earache, painful swellings and rheumatism: Chop 50g (2oz) or more of the whole plant and wrap it in muslin. Warm the parcel on a hot water bottle, radiator or hot tank. Hold it against the aching part. Warm it up when it cools and apply it again.

For a sore throat: Infuse 30ml (2 tablespoons) chopped flowers and leaves in 500ml (16floz) boiling water for 10 minutes. Strain. Use the infusion, hot, as a gargle and mouthwash four times a day, reheating it when necessary and gargling for 5–10 minutes at a time.

WILD MARJORAM, WILD THYME

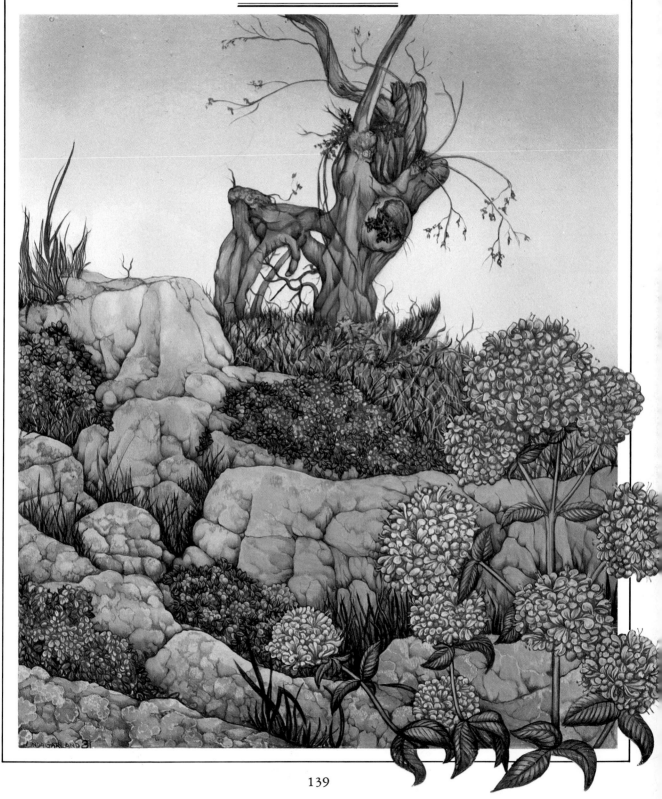

Availability

Wild thyme grows throughout Britain, Europe and Scandinavia. In the United States it is found mainly in the mid-west. In Australia it is not found in the wild but is very easy to grow.

It grows in dry, exposed places, on chalk cliffs and downs, banks, dunes and grassy heaths. It can be found on mountainsides and also in valleys where the soil is barren and stony. Other places to look are woodland clearings, by roadsides and on dry lawns.

Wild thyme is a perennial plant but it is not easy to find until the flowers appear. It blooms from mid-summer until early autumn (June to September in the northern hemisphere/December to March in Australasia).

Cut the small sprigs with scissors and use both the flowering tips and the leaves. The stems are usually too tough. Use wild thyme immediately or dry it for future use.

Courgettes (Zucchini) with Wild Thyme

This way of cooking courgettes (zucchini) preserves a light, fresh flavour.

450 g (1 lb) courgettes (zucchini)
25 g (1 oz) butter
30 ml (2 tablespoons) chopped wild thyme
juice ½ lemon

Coarsely grate the courgettes. Melt the butter in a saucepan on a high heat. Stir in the courgettes and wild thyme. Keep stirring until they begin to soften (about 2 minutes).

Pour in the lemon juice, let it bubble and take the pan from the heat. Serve as soon as possible. Serves 4.

Lambs Liver with Wild Thyme

Delicate herbs complement delicate flavours and wild thyme is perfect for liver.

675 g (1½ lbs) lamb's liver
40 g (1½ oz) wholewheat flour, seasoned
50 g (2 oz) butter
125 g (4 oz) mushrooms, thinly sliced
275 ml (½ pint) stock
45 ml (3 tablespoons) chopped wild thyme

Cut the liver into small, thin slices and coat them in the seasoned flour. Reserve any spare flour.

Melt 40 g (1½ oz) of the butter in a large frying pan on a high heat. Put in the pieces of liver, brown them on each side and remove them.

Lower the heat and melt the remaining butter in the pan. Put in the mushrooms and cook them for 1 minute. Stir in 15 ml (1 tablespoon) of the reserved flour. Pour in the stock and bring it to the boil, stirring. Put in the wild thyme and the liver and simmer, uncovered, for 5 minutes. Serves 4.

Wild Thyme Cheese with Tomato Salad

Wild thyme cheese can be eaten with bread or crackers, or it can be made into a first course with tomatoes.

45 ml (3 tablespoons) chopped wild thyme
225 g (8 oz) cream cheese
1 clove garlic, crushed with a pinch sea salt
freshly ground black pepper
4 large tomatoes
16 almonds
16 small parsley sprigs

Make sure the thyme is very finely chopped. Mix it into the cheese with the garlic and pepper.

Cut the tomatoes into four thick slices and arrange them on each of four small plates. Put a portion of the wild thyme cheese on each tomato slice and top each one with an almond and parsley sprig. Serves 4.

Shoulder of Lamb with Wild Thyme

As with the trout, wrapping lamb in a parcel with herbs subtly flavours it from the outside to the bone.

one half shoulder of lamb
2 cloves garlic
olive oil for greasing
sea salt and freshly ground black pepper
16 sprigs wild thyme
150 ml (¼ pint) dry white wine
150 ml (¼ pint) stock

Heat the oven to reg 4/180C/350F. Cut the garlic into very thin slivers. Cut slits in the lamb and insert the garlic.

Grease a large sheet of waxed paper with the oil. Season the paper well. Lay 8 sprigs of wild thyme on the paper and put the lamb on top. Cover the lamb with the remaining thyme sprigs and then wrap it up completely in the oiled paper. Wrap the parcel again in an ungreased piece of waxed paper and put it into a roasting tin. Roast the lamb for 2 hours.

Unwrap the parcel while it is still in the tin so you retain all the juices. Put the lamb onto a carving dish and if necessary, skim the juices. Put the tin with the juices on top of the stove on a high heat and pour in the wine and stock. Bring them to the boil and simmer for 1 minute.

Carve the lamb and serve the sauce separately. Serves 4.

Eggs in Snow with Wild Thyme

Wild thyme gives a delicate flavour to a light, airy dish of baked eggs.

4 eggs, separated
sea salt and white pepper
30 ml (2 tablespoons) chopped wild thyme
60 ml (4 tablespoons) thick cream
30 ml (2 tablespoons) grated Parmesan cheese

Heat the oven to Reg 8/230 C/450 F. Stiffly whip the egg whites. Fold in the salt and pepper with a metal spoon.

Pile the egg whites into a buttered, flat, oven-proof dish and in them make four evenly spaced depressions with the back of a spoon. Sprinkle a little wild thyme into each one.

Carefully tip an egg yolk into each depression. Spoon the cream round the edge of the yolks and scatter the Parmesan cheese over the whites.

Bake the eggs for 10 minutes, so the whites are risen and golden but the yolks are still slightly runny. Serve them directly from the dish, lifting out carefully with a spatula. Serves 4 as a light meal, 2 as a main meal.

Parcels of Trout with Wild Thyme

Cooked in parcels, trout become delicately permeated with the soft flavour of wild thyme.

4 trout
90 ml (6 tablespoons) chopped wild thyme
1 lemon
butter for greasing

Heat the oven to Reg 6/200 C/400 F. Clean the trout and cut off the heads. Make two diagonal slits downwards from head to tail on each side of the trout. Fill them with chopped wild thyme.

Cut all the rind and pith from the lemon and cut the flesh into lengthways quarters. Put a quarter inside each trout.

Wrap each trout separately in buttered aluminium foil and lay the parcels on a baking sheet. Bake the trout for 25 minutes.

To serve, unwrap each parcel separately onto an individual plate so as to catch all the juices. Serves 4.

Wild Thyme Scone

This light scone, delicately flavoured with wild thyme can be eaten hot or cold, with or without butter. If cold, it is best on the day that it is made. It is good with salads and with cheese.

225 g (8 oz) wholewheat flour
2.5 ml (½ teaspoon) sea salt
2.5 ml (½ teaspoon) bicarbonate of soda (baking soda)
40 g (1½ oz) lard
45 ml (3 tablespoons) chopped wild thyme
150 ml (¼ pint) natural yoghurt

Heat the oven to Reg 6/200 C/400 F. Put the flour into a bowl with the salt and soda. Rub in the lard, toss in the wild thyme. Make a well in the centre and pour in the yoghurt. Mix everything to a dough and knead it lightly.

Put the dough into a floured baking sheet and press it into a round 18 cm (7 inches) in diameter. Score the top into 12 triangles.

Bake the scone for 30 minutes so it is golden brown and risen.

Medicinal

To stimulate the circulation and tone the skin: Boil 500 g (1 lb) dried wild thyme in 4 litres (7 pints) water for 5 minutes. Take the pan from the heat and let the decoction stand for 10 minutes. Strain and add it to the bath water.

For a nervous headache: Infuse 15 ml (1 tablespoon) chopped wild thyme in 250 ml (8 fl oz) boiling water for 10 minutes. Strain, sweeten with honey if required, and drink the whole amount twice a day. Also, sniff thyme vinegar (made like mint vinegar page 116) like smelling salts.

For a hangover: Drink the above thyme infusion (as for nervous headache) three times a day.

A scalp tonic: Infuse 15 g (½ oz) dried wild thyme in 1 litre (1¾ pints) boiling water until cool. Strain. Rub a small amount into the scalp every day.

For catarrh and sore throat: Infuse 25 g (1 oz) dried wild thyme in 575 ml (1 pint) boiling water for 15 minutes. Strain and sweeten with honey. Take two tablespoons every two hours.

For whooping cough and bouts of fitful coughing: Boil 15 g (½ oz) dried wild thyme in 1 litre (1¾ pints) water until the liquid is reduced by half. Strain and sweeten with honey. Take 15 ml (1 tablespoon) every two hours after the start of the attack.

Veterinary

Bees love wild thyme so plant it near hives.
When goats and sheep eat wild thyme regularly both milk and meat will taste sweet.
For colic and pectoral ailments, boil a handful of the fresh herb in 1.15 litres (1½ pints) water for 3 minutes. Let the brew stand until cool and strain. Mix 250 ml (8 fl oz) of the brew into the feed morning and evening.

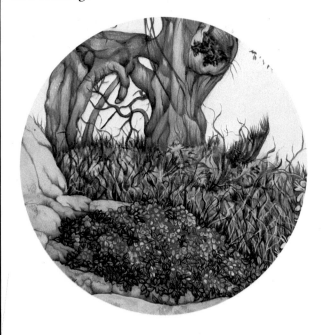

AUTUMN
FALL

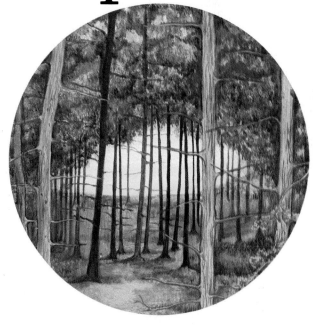

CHICORY

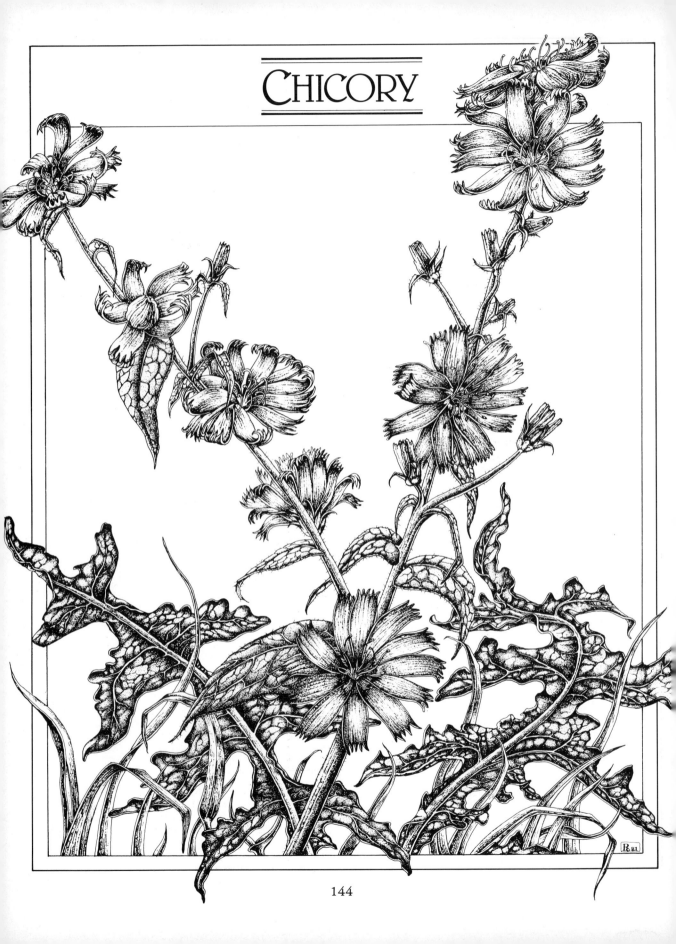

Availability

Chicory grows throughout Britain, Europe and Scandinavia, but it is more common in the south. It was introduced to the United States by European immigrants and now can mostly be found in the mid-western and southern states and Florida and to a certain extent along the Pacific coast.

Chicory thrives in very poor soil and can be found on the edges of fields, on waste ground and often by roadsides where the soil is so thin that it looks as though nothing could grow.

Pick the leaves in spring when they are young and tender (February to early April in the northern hemisphere). Pick them separately from the plant.

They will keep in a plastic bag in the bottom of the refrigerator for up to two days.

The flowers can be picked all through summer. Pick them in the morning while they are still open and use them as soon as possible to obtain the best effect for they will very quickly close.

The roots of chicory tend to become more brittle as they age, so dig them up in early autumn (September in the northern hemisphere), preferably just after it has rained so they are fairly pliable. They go down very deep so it is best to use a large spade.

Coffee Substitute

Roasted, ground chicory root added to ground coffee beans is said to counteract the over-stimulating effect that coffee can have on some people. If it is mixed with dandelion coffee (page 27) it will add extra flavour, making it more like real coffee. Chicory can also be used on its own as a coffee substitute. It has a strong, slightly bitter flavour so you will need to use less than you do real coffee.

Dig the roots of chicory, scrub them well and dry them. Cut them into 2.5 cm (1 inch) pieces and put them on a wire tray. Put them into a preheated Reg 3/170C/325F oven for about 2 hours so they become dry and dark brown. Cool them and grind them like coffee beans.

Add 10 ml (2 teaspoons) ground chicory to every 60 ml (4 tablespoons) dandelion coffee; and 5 ml (1 teaspoon) to every 60 ml (4 tablespoons) ground coffee beans.

To make a drink from all chicory, put 45 ml (3 tablespoons) ground chicory into a saucepan with 850 ml (1½ pints) water. Bring to the boil and simmer gently for 10 minutes. Strain into a warm jug and serve black or with milk and cream and sugar to taste as with ordinary coffee.

A garnish for salads

Pick chicory flowers when they are open and scatter them over green salads. They have a bitter flavour so use them sparingly and add a little honey to the dressing to balance the effect.

Green Salad with Chicory Leaves

1 round lettuce
50 g (2 oz) chicory leaves
½ medium sized cucumber
4 spring onions
60 ml (4 tablespoons) chopped chervil (or parsley)
10 ml (2 teaspoons) dill seeds
60 ml (4 tablespoons) olive oil
30 ml (2 tablespoons) white wine vinegar
5 ml (1 teaspoon) honey
freshly ground black pepper

Shred the lettuce and chicory leaves. Cut the cucumber into lengthways quarters and thinly slice them. Finely chop the spring onions.

Put the lettuce, chicory leaves, cucumber and spring onions into a bowl with the chervil (or parsley) and dill seeds. Beat the remaining ingredients together to make the dressing and fold them into the salad. Serves 4.

Bacon with Chicory Dressing

Chicory leaves can make a bitter-sharp, hot dressing for bacon.

125 g (4 oz) chicory leaves
1 medium onion
60 ml (4 tablespoons) white wine vinegar
10 ml (2 teaspoons) Dijon mustard
25 g (1 oz) pork dripping (or butter)
8 green back bacon rashers

Finely chop the chicory leaves. Quarter and thinly slice the onion. Beat the vinegar and mustard together. Fry the bacon rashers in the dripping or butter. Arrange them on a warm serving dish and keep them warm.

Pour all but 30 ml (2 teaspoons) fat from the pan and put it back on a medium heat. Put in the onion and stir it about until it begins to brown. Put in the chicory and keep stirring until it wilts (about 1 minute). Pour in the vinegar mixture, let it bubble and immediately spoon the contents of the pan over the bacon. Serves 4.

Medicinal

To restore appetite, tone the digestive system and combat anaemia: Eat the young leaves in a salad every day when they are at their best.
Or, boil 25 g (1 oz) chopped chicory root in 1 litre (1¾ pints) water for 15 minutes. Strain and take 225 ml (8 fl oz) before each of the three meals of the day.

For gallstones: Boil 10 ml (2 teaspoons) grated chicory root in 225 ml (8 fl oz) water for 2–3 minutes. Let it stand, covered, for 10 minutes and then strain off the liquid. Drink the whole amount twice a day.
Or, put 10 ml (2 teaspoons) dried chicory leaves into a saucepan with 225 ml (8 fl oz) water. Bring to the boil, take it from the heat and let it stand for 15 minutes. Strain. Take the whole amount, morning and evening, for six weeks.

For skin diseases, spots, eczema: Bring 15 g (½ oz) dried chicory leaves to the boil in 1 litre (1¾ pints) water. Take them from the heat and infuse, covered, for 10 minutes. Strain. Drink one cupful at meal times.

Veterinary

In Europe, chicory has been cultivated as a fodder crop which, as a fresh food, is highly nutritious to horses, cows and sheep, and is available when other green food is scarce. Chicory grows quickly and can be cut twice in the first year and three times for several years after. It does not, however, dry well and so is best not used for hay.
For general debility in cattle and all liver weakness including jaundice, give 50 g (2 oz) shredded root in a bran mash twice a day.

CEP

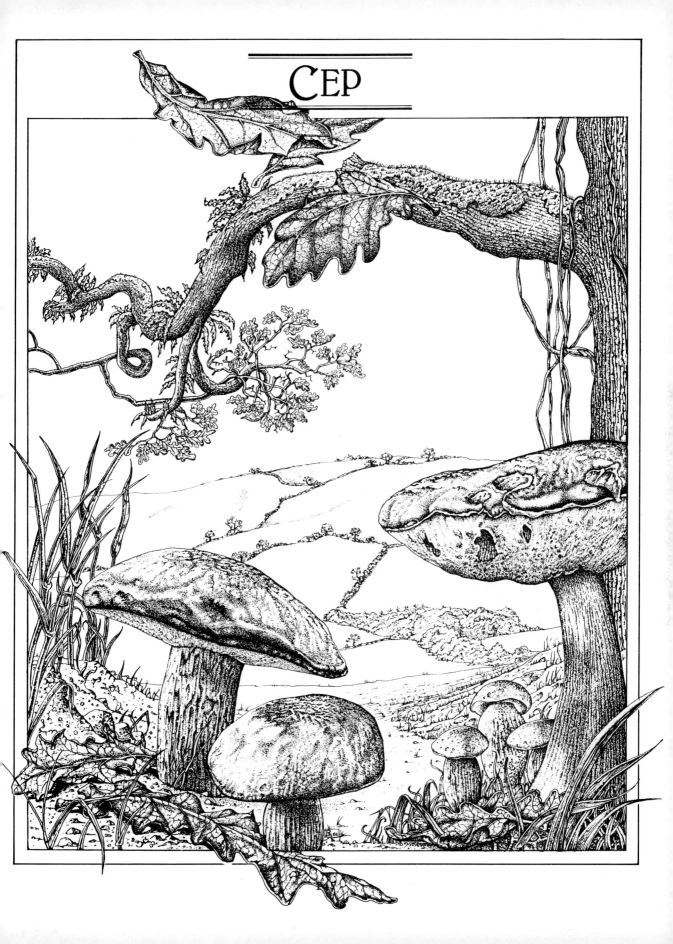

Availability

The cep grows throughout Britain, Europe, Scandinavia and the United States. It can be found in both deciduous and conifer woods and is particularly likely to grow where there are ancient pine trees and birch trees. It will spring up under trees, on the edges of woods and very often near woodland paths.

Ceps can be found all through summer but are most abundant in the autumn (late August to early November in the northern hemisphere). You are most likely to find them when the weather has been damp but not exceptionally wet.

Whilst hunting for ceps, you will probably find other varieties of Boletus mushroom which can be used in the same ways. In Britain, Scandinavia and Europe look for Boletus badius, subtomentosus, chrysenteron, luteus, scaber and testeoscaber. In the United States the other edible varieties of Boletus are chromapes, mirabilis, affinis, russellii, chrysenteron, bicolor, pallidus and badius. Always take field guides out with you and know what you are looking for.

Ceps are best to eat when they are dry and from 3 cm to 10 cm (1½ to 4 inches) across, as you can cook or dry the caps whole. However do not leave the large ones behind. If any parts of them look soggy, cut them out immediately after picking.

Twist all Boletus mushrooms out of the ground. Cut off the end of the stipe with a sharp knife and leave it on the ground near to where you found the mushroom. Always carry ceps in an open basket.

Preparing Ceps for Cooking

If the mushrooms are small and firm, all you need do is thinly slice them. Watch out for insects, however, and cut any inhabited parts away. The stipes are also edible. Thinly slice them. If the tubes on the underside of the caps are soggy, cut them away and discard them, otherwise, they will make your final dish rather watery.

When weighing for a particular recipe, weigh after preparing.

Ceps in Soured Cream

Quick cooking ensures that the ceps stay firm and tasty. The amounts given here will serve four as a side dish with a main meal. They are rich and filling so you only need small amounts. As a snack meal for two serve the mushrooms on wholemeal toast, two slices per person, and top them with chopped parsley.

225 g (8 oz) ceps (prepared weight)
25 g (1 oz) butter
30 ml (2 tablespoons) soured cream
30 ml (2 tablespoons) lemon juice
freshly ground black pepper

Thinly slice the ceps. Melt the butter in frying pan on a high heat. Put in the ceps and stir them around for 2 minutes.

Add the soured cream and lemon juice and season liberally with pepper. Mix well and take the pan from the heat. Serve immediately.

Wild Mushroom Tartlets

These will make a snack meal for four people or a first course for six.

shortcrust pastry made with 175 g (6 oz) wholewheat flour
175 g (6 oz) ceps (prepared weight)
25 g (1 oz) butter
30 ml (2 tablespoons) soured cream
juice ½ lemon
freshly ground black pepper
12 very small parsley sprigs

Line twelve tartlet tins with the pastry. Bake them blind for 15 minutes in a preheated Reg 6/200C/400F oven. Keep them warm.

Finely chop the ceps and then cook them as above. Fill the tarlet cases with the mixture and top each one with a parsley sprig.

To Grill Ceps

For grilling, use only small, firm ceps. (Reserve the stipes for drying or for flavouring soups and casseroles).

Preheat the grill to the highest temperature. Brush the caps on both sides with melted butter. Lay them, underside up, on the hot grill rack and grill them, without turning, for three minutes, so they are cooked through and sizzling.

Just before serving, squeeze a little lemon juice over them.

Beef Skirt with Dried Ceps

This is a very rich dish. Serve it with creamed potatoes and a lightly cooked green vegetable.

675 g (1½ lbs) beef skirt, in two thin, flat pieces
   of even shape
50 g (2oz) dried ceps
575 ml (1 pint) stock, boiling
stuffing:
25 g (1 oz) butter
5 ml (1 teaspoon) dill seeds
50 g (2oz) breadcrumbs
60 ml (4 tablespoons) dry red wine
freshly ground black pepper
4 spring onions
for braising:
15 g (½ oz) butter
15 ml (1 tablespoon) wholewheat flour
200 ml (7 fl oz) mushroom stock
150 ml (¼ pint) dry red wine

Put the mushrooms into a bowl. Pour in the boiling stock and leave them for 1 hour. Drain them, reserving the stock, and finely chop them.

Heat the oven to Reg 4/180C/350F. For the stuffing, melt the butter in a small frying pan on a low heat. Put in half the mushrooms and the dill seeds and cook them gently for 5 minutes. Take the pan from the heat and mix in the breadcrumbs and wine. Season with the pepper.

Spread the stuffing over one piece of beef. Trim the spring onions to the same length as the beef and lay them on top of the stuffing in alternate directions. Lay the other piece of meat on top and tie the pieces together with fine cotton string, both crossways and lengthways.

To braise the beef, melt the butter in a flame-proof casserole on a high heat. Put in the beef, brown it on both sides and remove it. Lower the heat and put in the remaining mushrooms. Cook them for 2 minutes, stirring occasionally.

Dust in the flour and stir until it browns. Stir in the stock and wine and bring them to the boil. Put in the beef. Cover the casserole and put it into the oven for 1½ hours.

To serve, lift out the beef. Remove the string and cut the meat crossways into four pieces. Put them onto individual plates and spoon any sauce remaining in the casserole over the top. Serves 4.

To Dry Ceps

When you have a large crop of ceps, it is best to dry some for future use. Keep the smaller caps and stipes whole. Cut away any soggy parts from the larger caps. You may sometimes have to cut away all the tubes (the yellow parts underneath which look like sponge) if they are very wet. Cut the larger caps into pieces 4—5 cm (1½—2 inches) square. Cut the stipes into 6 cm (2½ inch) lengths.

Preheat the oven to Reg under ¼/70C/200F. Lay the pieces of mushroom on wire racks and put them into the oven for 30–40 minutes. They should still give slightly when you press them with your finger but should be quite dry. Take them out and cool them.

Thread a stout needle with a very long piece of strong cotton thread. Double the thread and tie a knot in the end. Tie the end round a piece of twig about 10 cm (4 inches) long, and then thread the pieces of mushroom onto the thread. When the mushrooms are about 15 cm (6 inches) deep, make a loop in the needle end of the thread. Hang the strings of mushrooms up by the loop. The stipes should be hung separately. Do not add them to cooked dishes but use them tied in bouquets garnis to give flavour to soups and casseroles.

Mushroom Powder

Put several pieces of dried mushroom cap or stipe into a blender, food processor or clean coffee grinder and grind them to a fine powder. Add just 5 ml (1 teaspoon) per 275 ml (½ pint) liquid before cooking to flavour soups and casseroles.

To Reconstitute Dried Ceps

Put the ceps into a bowl and pour on boiling water or stock. Leave them for 1 hour. Take them out, chop them and use them as cultivated mushrooms in recipes. They will have a much richer flavour than the same variety of mushroom used fresh.

25 g (1 oz) dried ceps will weigh about 75 g (3 oz) when reconstituted.

CRAB APPLE

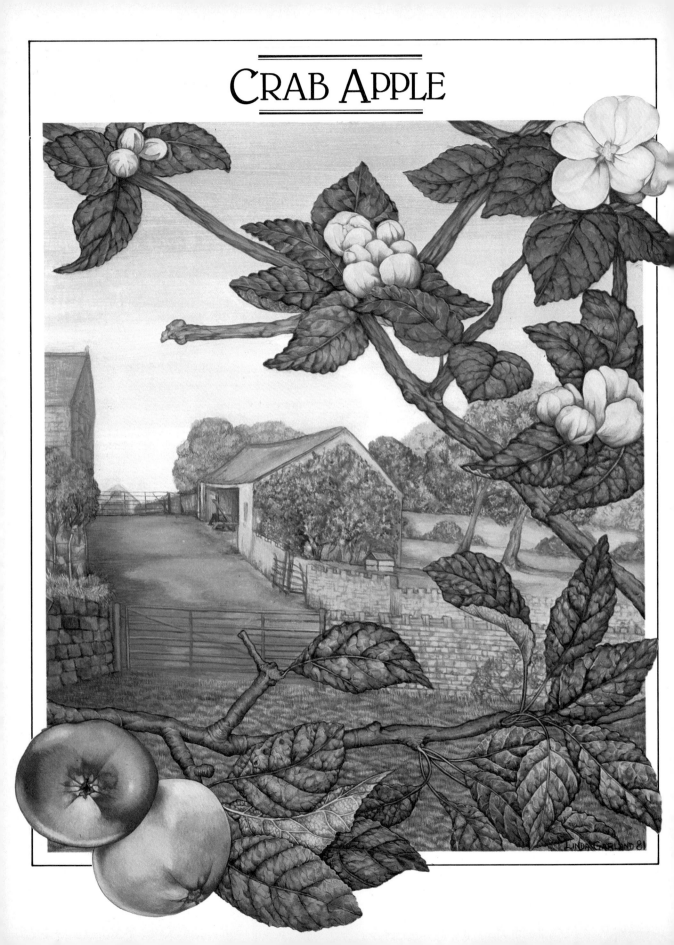

Availability

Crab apple trees grow throughout Britain and the temperate areas of Europe. They are rare in Scotland and will not grow at all in the hot climate of southern Europe.

Crab apple trees can be found in woods, along hedgerows and on exposed heathland. They can also be successfully cultivated both for decoration and for the fruits which can be used in the same ways as wild crab apples.

There are five related species in the United States. The narrow leaved crab apple (Pyrus angustifolia) grows in woods and thickets in the eastern, mid-western and southern states. The American crab apple (Malus glaucescens) can be found in the mid-western and eastern states in woods and also by roadsides. In the mid-western, southern plains states and the south can be found the western crab apple (Pyrus ioensis); and throughout the western states the Oregon crab apple (Pyrus diversifolia). The wilding tree, (Pyrus malus or Malus malus) grows in the north eastern states.

Crab apples can be picked from late summer to autumn (August to October in the northern hemisphere) but are best after the first frost. This mellows them and makes them softer and gives them a slightly translucent appearance.

Spiced Apple Butter

This apple butter is a dark brown colour due to the dark sugar and it tastes sweet, spiced and fruity.

Spread it over cakes, pile it into tarts, stir it into yoghurt or spoon it on top of ice cream.

1.8 kg (4 lbs) crab apples
1.15 litres (2 pints) water
15 ml (1 tablespoon) whole cloves
2 chips nutmeg
two 5 cm (2 inch) pieces cinnamon stick
about 1.125 kg (2½ lbs) dark brown (Barbados) sugar

Halve the crab apples and put them into a preserving pan with the water, cloves, nutmeg and cinnamon. Bring them to the boil and simmer them, stirring occasionally, for about 1 hour, so they can be beaten to a thick pulp.

Put the pulp through the fine blade of a vegetable mill and weigh it. Return it to the cleaned preserving pan and stir in 350 g (12 oz) sugar for every 450 g (1 lb) apple purée.

Set the pan on a low heat and stir for the sugar to dissolve. Bring to the boil and keep boiling, stirring frequently, until the butter is very thick. If you draw a wooden spoon through it it should leave a path behind it. This may take up to one hour.

Put the butter into warmed preserving jars and cover it tightly while it is still hot. The butter will be ready for use as soon as it is cool. Once a jar has been opened, store it in the refrigerator.

Fills about four and a half 450 g (1 lb) jars.

Pork Chops with Crab Apple Crust

Crab apples mixed with sage, onions and wholewheat breadcrumbs make a colourful crusty top for pork chops.

4 loin pork chops
12 sage leaves
225 g (8 oz) crab apples
1 medium onion, finely chopped
50 g (2 oz) fresh wholewheat breadcrumbs
freshly ground black pepper

Heat the oven to Reg 6/200C/400F. Cut the rind from the chops, leaving most of the fat. Put the chops on a rack in a roasting tin and put the rinds into the tin to render down. Lay two sage leaves on each chop and put the chops into the oven for 45 minutes.

While the chops are cooking, finely chop the remaining sage leaves and quarter, core and finely chop the crab apples. Spoon 45 ml (3 tablespoons) fat from the roasting tin into a small frying pan. Set the pan on a low heat, mix in the onion and crab apples and cook them until the onion is soft. Take the pan from the heat and mix in the breadcrumbs, sage and pepper.

Spread the stuffing mixture over the lean part only of the chops, leaving the fat to crisp. Return the chops to the oven for a further 15 minutes for the crust to brown. Serve the chops plainly, with no sauce or gravy. Serves 4.

Lamb with Crab Apple Stuffing

The sharpness of crab apples in a stuffing goes well with rich meats like lamb.

one joint best end neck lamb weighing 750–850g (1½–1¾lbs) with bones
75g (3oz) crab apples
15g (½oz) butter
1 small onion, finely chopped
1 clove garlic, finely chopped
50g (2oz) fresh wholewheat breadcrumbs
5ml (1 teaspoon) chopped rosemary
60ml (4 tablespoons) dry cider

Heat the oven to Reg 6/200C/400F. Bone the lamb (or get your butcher to do it for you). Quarter, core and finely chop the crab apples.

Melt the butter in a frying pan on a low heat. Put in the onion and garlic and soften them. Take the pan from the heat and mix in the breadcrumbs, rosemary, crab apples and cider.

Put the stuffing on the cut surface of the lamb. Roll up the lamb and tie it in about six places with fine cotton string. Put it on a rack in a roasting tin and put it into the oven for 1 hour. Cut the lamb into eight slices for serving. Serves 4.

Crab Apple and Date Wine

This is a pinky-amber coloured, rich, fruity wine.

2.25kg (5lbs) crab apples
900g (2lbs) pressed dates
1.15kg (2½lbs) sugar
4.6 litres (1 gallon) boiling water
juice 4 lemons
225ml (8floz) strong cold black tea
yeast
yeast nutrient
pectolase

Pick over the crab apples and discard the stalks. Put the crab apples into a plastic container and mash them to a pulp. Chop the dates and add them to the crab apples. Mix in the sugar. Pour the boiling water onto the fruits, stir well and cool to lukewarm.

Add the lemon juice, tea, yeast, yeast nutrient and pectolase. Leave the brew, covered, for five days in a warm place, stirring every day.

Strain the liquid into a 4.6 litre (1 gallon) jar and fit a fermentation lock. Rack as the wine clears and bottle it when fermentation is complete. Leave the wine for at least nine months before opening.

Crab Apple Cake

This moist, spicy cake rises round the crab apples so that by the time it comes out of the oven they are set into the top. Serve it as a dessert, rather than a tea time cake.

350g (12oz) crab apples
45ml (3 tablespoons) honey
5ml (1 teaspoon) ground cinnamon
base:
225g (8oz) wholewheat flour
pinch sea salt
5ml (1 teaspoon) bicarbonate of soda
125g (4oz) butter
125g (4oz) light brown (demerara) sugar
150ml (¼ pint) natural yoghurt

Heat the oven to Reg 6/200C/400F. Quarter, core and chop the crab apples. Mix them in a bowl with the honey and cinnamon.

Put the flour into a bowl with the salt, bicarbonate of soda and cinnamon. Rub in the butter. Toss in the sugar with your fingertips. Make a well in the centre, pour in the yoghurt and mix everything to a moist dough.

Put the mixture into a buttered, 5cm (2 inch) deep and 20 by 25cm (8 by 10 inch) tin. Cover the top with the crab apples. Bake the cake for 30 minutes so the top browns and a skewer inserted in the centre comes out clean. Serve it hot, with cream. Serves 6.

Crab Apple Pudding

To make a purée of crab apples, simply chop them, skins and cores included, cook them and rub them through a sieve.

A sweet, spiced crab apple purée can be topped with an oatmeal and flour cake mixture to make a warming autumn pudding.

450g (1lb) crab apples
150ml (¼ pint) water
50g (2oz) light brown (Barbados) sugar
pinch ground cloves
top:
125g (4oz) wheatmeal self raising flour
25g (4oz) medium oatmeal
125g (4oz) light brown (Barbados) sugar
pinch ground cloves
125g (4oz) butter
2 eggs, beaten
60ml (4 tablespoons) milk

Heat the oven to Reg 4/180C/350F. Chop the crab apples and put them into a saucepan with the water. Set them on a low heat. Cover them and cook them for about 25 minutes, stirring occasionally. You should be able to beat them to a thick purée. Rub the purée through a sieve and stir in the sugar and ground cloves.

Make the top while the apples are cooking. In a bowl, mix together the flour, oatmeal, sugar and cloves. Make a well in the centre. Melt the butter and pour it into the flour. Add the eggs and milk and beat with a wooden spoon until you have a smooth mixture.

Put the crab apple purée into a large, buttered pie dish. Cover it with the pudding mixture. Bake the pudding for 30 minutes so it is golden brown and firm. Serve it hot, with cream. Serves 4.

Individual Crab Apple Crumbles

Crab apples can be made into crumble puddings in the same way as large cooking apples. Quarter and core them only. There is no need to peel them. Muesli base makes a light crumbly topping which makes a change from the more conventional one made with flour, butter and sugar.

450 g (1 lb) crab apples
150 g (5 oz) ground cinnamon
60 ml (4 tablespoons) honey
crumble:
175 g (6 oz) muesli base
60 ml (4 tablespoons) sesame seeds
60 ml (4 tablespoons) desiccated coconut
60 ml (4 tablespoons) sunflower oil

Heat the oven to Reg 6/200C/400F. Core and chop the crab apples. Put them into a bowl and mix in the sultanas, cinnamon and honey. Divide the apples between four small heatproof bowls.

Mix together the muesli base, sesame seeds, coconut and oil. Divide them between the bowls, covering the crab apples completely. Bake the crumbles for 25 minutes so the tops are golden brown. They are best eaten hot with cream, soured cream or natural yoghurt, but they are also very good cold. Serves 4.

DAMSON

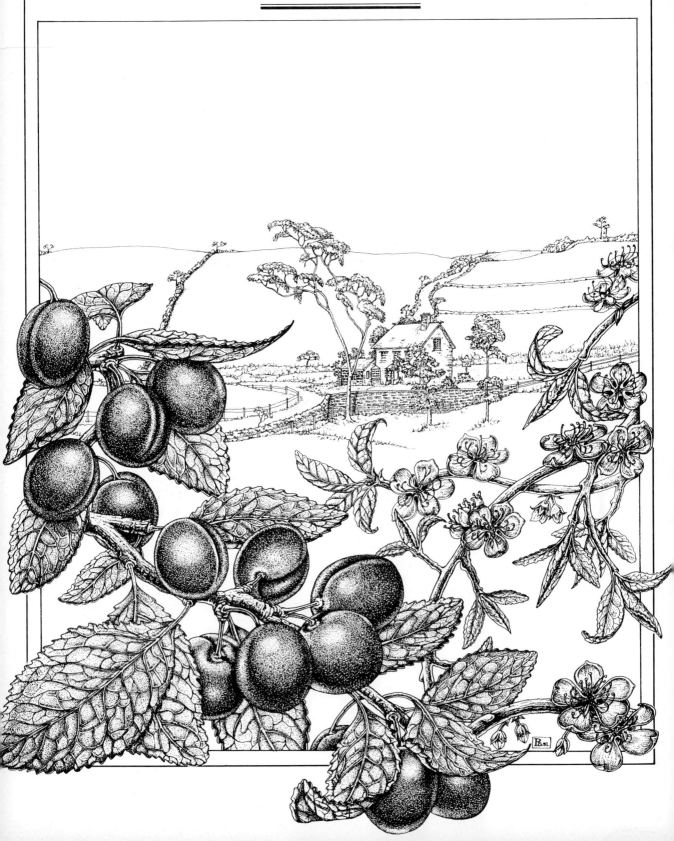

Availability

Damsons were originally found in the Middle East by the crusaders who took them back to Britain and Europe where they can now be found both cultivated and growing wild. You can find wild damson trees in woods and thickets and along hedgerows and also on the sites of abandoned orchards.

The fruits can be picked in early autumn (September and the beginning of October in the northern hemisphere). They will keep for five days in a cool place if you are unable to use them straight away.

The bullace or wild plum (Prunus insititia) is closely related to the damson and has a similar, dry spicy flavour. Where the damson has a slightly oval shape, the bullace is round, often up to 2.5 cm (1 inch) across. Both are a deep purple colour with a lighter bloom. Bullaces can be substituted for damsons in all the recipes below.

In the United States, the Sierra (Pacific or Californian) Plum (Prunus subcordata) is the most similar fruit. Although dark red in colour it has the same acid flavour and the flesh clings to the stone like that of damsons. It can be found on the west coast from south Oregon and all through western California. Other American species which can be substituted are the beach plum (Prunus maritima) which grows on sea beaches and sand dunes, mainly in the eastern states; and the Chickasaw plum (Prunus angustifolia) which can be found in the eastern and southern states. The Chickasaw plum is best for preserving.

Pork Tenderloin with Damsons

Pork fillet cooked with damsons becomes pinky brown and the damsons make a slightly pink, translucent sauce.

675–900 g (1½–2lbs) pork tenderloin
1 clove garlic, finely chopped
pinch sea salt
8 black peppercorns
4 juniper berries
4 allspice berries
175 g (6 oz) damsons
275 ml (½ pint) dry cider

Heat the oven to Reg 6/200C/400F. Cut the pork into four even sized pieces. Slit each piece open, keeping it joined down one side. Lay the pieces out flat, cut side up. Crush the garlic, salt, peppercorns, juniper berries and allspice berries together and spread them evenly over the surface of the pork. Halve and stone the damsons and arrange them evenly over one side of each of the pork pieces. Fold the pork back into shape and tie it with strong cotton thread.

Put the pork pieces into an ovenproof casserole in a single layer and pour in the cider. Cover the casserole and put it into the oven for 1 hour.

Lift out the pork pieces and remove the thread. Arrange the pork on a warmed serving dish. Bring the juices in the casserole to simmering point and pour them over the pork. Serves 4.

Pot Roast Lamb with Damsons

Damsons make a rich, fruity sauce for a pot roast of lamb.

225 g (8 oz) damsons
one shoulder lamb
2 sprigs lemon thyme
3 sprigs marjoram
15 g (½ oz) butter
1 small onion, thinly sliced
275 ml (½ pint) stock

Heat the oven to Reg 4/180C/350F. Halve and stone the damsons. Bone the lamb. Chop the leaves of one sprig of each of the herbs and scatter them over the cut surface of the meat. Roll up the lamb and tie it with fine cotton string.

Melt the butter in a flameproof casserole on a high heat. Put in the lamb and brown it all over. Remove it. Lower the heat. Put in the onion and soften it. Pour in the stock, add the damsons and bring the stock to the boil. Put in the lamb and the remaining herb sprigs. Cover the casserole and put it into the oven for 1 hour 3o minutes.

Take out the lamb and keep it warm. Skim the fruity juices in the casserole and then rub them through a sieve to make the sauce. Reheat it. Carve the lamb and serve the sauce separately. Serves 6.

Lamb Chops Baked with Damsons

Again the sauce made by the damsons is rich and fruity and an attractive deep red.

8 small loin lamb chops
freshly grated nutmeg
225 g (8 oz) damsons
1 medium onion, finely chopped
1 clove garlic, finely chopped
5 cm (2 inch) piece cinnamon stick
60 ml (4 tablespoons) red wine vinegar

Heat the oven to Reg 6/200C/400F. Trim any excess fat from the chops and grate some nutmeg over both sides. Halve and stone the damsons, put them into a flat, ovenproof dish with the garlic, cinnamon, stock and wine vinegar. Put the chops on top.

Put the dish into the oven for 50 minutes, turning the chops once. Take out the chops and put them into a warmed serving dish. Remove the cinnamon stick and skim the damsons if necessary. Spoon them over the chops to serve. Serves 4.

Damson and Date Pie

Sharp damsons definitely benefit from the additional sweetness of a dried fruit and the cinnamon completes the rich pie filling which has a flavour reminiscent of mulled wine.

shortcrust pastry made with 225 g (8 oz) wholewheat
    flour
350 g (12 oz) damsons
50 g (2 oz) stoned dried dates
125 g (4 oz) dark brown (Barbados) sugar
2.5 ml (½ teaspoon) ground cinnamon
beaten egg or milk to glaze

Heat the oven to Reg 6/200C/400F. Make the pastry and chill it for a short time. Halve and stone the damsons and finely chop the dates. Put them together in a bowl and mix in the sugar and cinnamon.

Line a 20 cm (8 inch) enamel pie plate with about two thirds of the pastry. Put in the damson filling and cover it with the remaining pastry. Seal the edges and use any pastry scraps to decorate the top.

Brush the pie with beaten egg or milk and bake it for 25 minutes so the top is golden brown. Serve the pie hot or cold. Serves 4.

Green Pepper and Damsons

Savoury peppers and sharp damsons make an unusual accompaniment for pork, lamb or oily fish.

4 medium sized green peppers
225 g (8 oz) damsons
45 ml (3 tablespoons) olive oil
1 large onion, thinly sliced
1 clove garlic, finely chopped

Core and deseed the peppers and cut them into pieces 2.5 cm by 6 mm (1 inch by ¼ inch). Halve and stone the damsons. Heat the oil in a large frying pan on a low heat. Put in the onion and garlic and soften them.

Mix in the peppers and cook them until the onions are brown, stirring occasionally. Add the damsons and let them heat through and begin to "bleed" a light crimson colour. Serve as soon as possible so they stay whole. Serves 4.

Damson and Apple Cobbler

This is a warming autumn pudding.

top:
175 g (6 oz) wholewheat flour
10 ml (2 teaspoons) caraway seeds
2.5 ml (½ teaspoon) ground cinnamon
2.5 ml (½ teaspoon) baking powder
100 g (3½ oz) lard
50 g (2 oz) light brown (demerara) sugar
2 eggs, beaten
filling:
225 g (8 oz) damsons
350 g (12 oz) cooking apples
pinch ground cloves
125 g light brown (demerara) sugar

Heat the oven to Reg 4/180C/350F. Put the flour into a bowl with the caraway seeds, cinnamon and baking powder and rub in the lard as though you are making pastry. Toss in the sugar. Make a well in the centre and gradually mix in the eggs. Beat the mixture with a wooden spoon to make it smooth.

Halve and stone the damsons. Peel, core and slice the apples. Put them together in a bowl and mix in the cloves and sugar. Put the damson and apple mixture into a 23 or 25 cm (9 or 10 inch) diameter flan dish and spread the cobbler mixture evenly over the top. Bake the cobbler for 35 minutes so the top is golden brown. Serve the cobbler hot, with cream, soured cream or natural yoghurt. Serves 6.

Damson and Orange Pie

Damsons, orange and mace make a rich, dark filling with an old fashioned flavour for a pie.

pastry:
225 g (8 oz) wholewheat flour
5 ml (1 teaspoon) baking powder
pinch sea salt
50 g (2 oz) lard
75 g (3 oz) butter
60 ml (4 tablespoons) cold water
beaten egg for glaze
filling:
450 g (1 lb) damsons
grated rind and juice 1 large orange
pinch ground mace
60 ml (4 tablespoons) honey
30 ml (2 tablespoons) tapioca or sago

Make the pastry and leave it in a cool place. Stone the damsons and put them into a saucepan with the orange rind and juice, mace and honey. Set them on a low heat, cover them and cook them for 15 minutes so they become very juicy. Take the pan from the heat and mix in the tapioca or sago. Leave the damsons until they are completely cold.

Heat the oven to Reg 6/200C/400F. Roll out two thirds of the pastry and use it to line an 18 cm (7 inch) diameter 4 cm (2 inch) deep pie plate. Put in the damsons and cover them with the remaining pastry. Seal the edges and brush the pie with beaten egg. Bake the pie for 30 minutes so it is golden brown. Serve it hot or cold with soured cream, natural yoghurt or whipped cream.
Serves 6.

Spiced Damson Jelly

Serve this dark red jelly with roast lamb or game.

900 g (2 lbs) damsons
150 ml (¼ pint) water
275 ml (½ pint) red wine vinegar
10 ml (2 teaspoons) black peppercorns
10 ml (2 teaspoons) allspice berries
2 dried red chillies
about 350 g (12 oz) light brown (demerara) sugar

Slit the damsons all round with a sharp knife and put them into a saucepan with the water, vinegar and spices. Bring them gently to the boil and simmer them for 40 minutes so you have a very juicy pulp.

Strain the pulp through a jelly bag. Measure the juice and return it to the cleaned pan. Stir in 450 g (1 lb) sugar to every 575 ml (1 pint) juice. Stir until the sugar has dissolved and bring it to the boil. Boil until setting point is reached.

Pour the jelly into warmed jars and cover it with circles of waxed paper. Cover it completely when cold. Makes about 450 g (1 lb).

Damson and Raisin Chutney

This is a rich, dark chutney. Serve it with cold lamb or beef, ham and cheese.

1.35 kg (3 lbs) damsons
450 g (1 lb) raisins, finely chopped
275 ml (½ pint) red wine vinegar
175 g (6 oz) dark brown (Barbados) sugar
15 ml (1 tablespoon) mustard seeds
5 ml (1 teaspoon) ground allspice

Stone the damsons and put them into a preserving pan with the rest of the ingredients. Bring them slowly to the boil and simmer them gently for 1 hour, stirring occasionally. The mixture should be very thick.

Pour the chutney into warm jars and cover it while it is still warm. Keep it for a month before opening. Unopened, it will keep for up to two years. Makes about 1.35 kg (3 lbs).

Damson Wine

This is a rich, red wine.

2.7 kg (6 lbs) damsons
1.575 kg (3 lbs) sugar
4.6 litres (1 gallon) boiling water
pectolase
juice 4 lemons
yeast
yeast nutrient

Stalk and wash the damsons. Put them into a container with 900 g (2 lbs) of the sugar. Pour on to the boiling water and stir well. Add the pectolase and cool to lukewarm.

Stir in the lemon juice, yeast and yeast nutrient and cover. Leave the brew to ferment in a warm place for five days, stirring every day.

Strain the liquid onto a syrup made from the remaining sugar and 425 ml (¾ pint) water. Put the mixture into a 4.6 litre (1 gallon) jar and fit a fermentation lock.

Rack as the wine clears and bottle it when fermentation is complete. Leave the wine for at least six months before opening.

ELDER

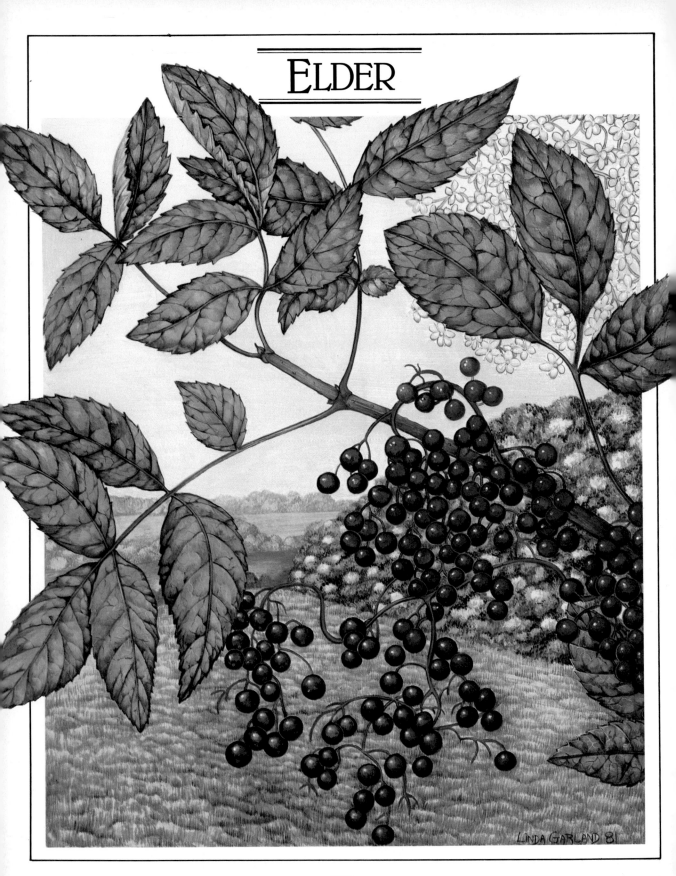

LINDA GARLAND 81

SAMBUCUS NIGRA

Local Names: Black Elder, Boon Tree, Bore Tree, Borral,
Bour Tree, Bull Tree, Common Elder, Devil's Wood, Dog Tree,
Eldern, Eller, Ellet, Judas Tree, Pipe Tree, Scaw, Scawen,
Tea-tree, Trammon, Whit Aller

Availability

The elder tree grows throughout Britain, Europe and Scandinavia. It can be found in woods and on scrub and waste ground, very often near the walls of derelict cottages. Hedgerows often have elder trees growing in them, particularly if there are rabbit warrens underneath.

There are two related species in the United States. The American or sweet elder (Sambucus canadensis), sometimes called Elderblow, grows in the mid-western and eastern states, the plains states and Texas. It is generally taller in the south than in the north. The blue berried elder (Sambucus glauca) is a much taller tree with larger and juicier berries. It grows mainly in the extreme western states and is cultivated as an ornamental tree along the Pacific coast.

The elder tree sports its creamy white, umbrella like clusters of tiny flowers all through early summer (May to July in the northern hemisphere). Medicinally, they are best picked just before they are fully open. Pick the whole flower heads either by hand or with scissors and either use them as soon as possible or dry them on muslin covered racks. Make sure, when picking the flowers, that you leave enough sprigs behind to give you plenty of fruits in the autumn.

If the leaves are needed for medicinal purposes, gather them on a fine morning in early summer after the dew has dried.

Elder berries are ready for picking in early autumn (September to October in the northern hemisphere). Ideally you should wait until the stems are a deep, pinky red and the clusters of berries are hanging downwards, but in waiting you may sacrifice a few to the birds. Some parts of the tree may ripen earlier than others. If this is the case it is best to visit the tree twice. When the berries are ripe the sprigs can easily be broken off by hand. Bend any tall branches towards you with the crook of a walking stick but be careful as they are brittle.

Use elder berries as soon as possible. To prepare them for cooking, strip them from the sprigs with a fork in the same way as you would red or black currants.

Elderberry Sauce

Serve this hot, sweet sauce with hot or cold roast beef or lamb; or with plainly cooked lamb chops.

350 g (12 oz) elderberries, weighed on stems
200 ml (7 fl oz) red wine vinegar
175 g (6 oz) dark brown (Barbados) sugar
1 large onion, finely chopped
10 ml (2 teaspoons) ground black pepper
5 ml (1 teaspoon) juniper berries, crushed
3 cm (1 inch) piece root ginger, bruised
1 chip nutmeg
1 dried red chilli

Remove the elderberries from the stems. Put them into a saucepan with the rest of the ingredients. Set them on a low heat until the juices begin to run.

Turn the heat up a little and bring the contents of the pan to the boil. Boil them gently for 1 hour so the juices become very thick.

Put the sauce through the fine blade of a vegetable mill or rub it through a sieve. Put it into a warm jar and cover it while it is still warm. Makes about 200 ml (7 fl oz).

Elderberry Turnovers

Elderberries make a fruity filling for turnovers that melts and bubbles like jam.

shortcrust pastry made with 225 g (8 oz) wholewheat flour
125 g (4 oz) elderberries (weighed when on stem)
30 ml (2 tablespoons) honey
little freshly grated nutmeg
beaten egg or milk for glaze

Heat the oven to Reg 6/200C/400F. Take the elderflowers off the sprigs and mix them with honey and nutmeg. Divide the pastry into six pieces and roll each one into a 12–15 cm (5–6 inch) triangle. Put a small portion of the elderberries on one side of each triangle. Fold over the other side and seal the edges.

Put the turnovers onto a floured baking sheet and brush them with beaten egg or milk. Bake them for 20 minutes or until they are golden brown. Serve them hot with cream or leave them until they are quite cold and pack them into a lunch box. Makes 6.

Elderflower Fritters with Gooseberry Purée

Elderflowers, just out of the bud stage, make delicate flavoured fritters. From bud to full-blown flower, the sprigs can give the subtle flavour of muscat grapes to gooseberries. In the United States where green gooseberries may not be available, greengages or green plums may be used instead. Halve and stone them before cooking.

fritters:
4 sprigs elderflowers
75 g (3 oz) wholewheat flour
pinch salt
2 eggs
15 ml (1 tablespoon) olive oil
90 ml (6 tablespoons) dry white wine
purée:
450 g (1 lb) green gooseberries
90 ml (6 tablespoons) dry white wine
1 elderflower sprig
30 ml (2 tablespoons) honey, or, to taste

First, make the batter. Put the flour and salt into a bowl. Make a well in the centre and beat in the eggs, one at a time. Beat in the oil and then the wine to make a fairly thick batter. Leave it to stand while you make the purée.

Put the gooseberries, whole, into a saucepan with the wine and elderflower sprig. Cover them and set them on a low heat for 15 minutes so they are very soft. Rub them through a sieve. Return the purée to the cleaned pan and stir in the honey. Stir on a low heat for it to dissolve. Keep the purée warm.

Heat a pan of deep oil to 170C/325F. Hold the stalk of the elderflower sprigs and dip the whole flower head into the batter. Deep fry the sprigs so they are crisp and golden brown. Drain them on kitchen paper.

Serve the fritters hot and have the gooseberry purée in a separate bowl to spoon over them. Serves 4.

Elderflower Vinegar

This vinegar gives a light, delicate flavour to lettuce, cucumber and corn salads.

one 500 ml (17.5 fl oz) bottle white wine vinegar
75 g (3 oz) elderflower sprigs

Put the elderflowers into a jar and pour in the vinegar. Seal the jar tightly and leave it on a sunny windowsill for 1 week. Strain the vinegar and bottle it.

Elderberry Rob

Elderberry Rob should really only be kept for medicinal purposes, but it makes a delicious warming drink on a cold night. Dilute it with three parts of hot water.

1.8 kg (4 lbs) elderberries, weighed on stem
two 5 cm (2 inch) pieces cinnamon stick
1 piece ginger root, bruised
2 chips nutmeg
5 ml (1 teaspoon) allspice berries
5 ml (1 teaspoon) cloves
275 ml (½ pint) water
350 g (12 oz) honey to each 575 ml (1 pint) liquid
150 ml (¼ pint) brandy

Take the elderberries from the stalks. Put them into a saucepan with the spices and water. Bring them gently to the boil and simmer them until the pan is full of juice, about 20 minutes.

Put a piece of muslin or an old linen tea towel over a large bowl. Pour the elderberries through it. Gather the sides together and squeeze out as much juice as you can. Measure it and return it to the cleaned saucepan.

Bring the juice to the boil and add the honey. Stir for it to dissolve and then boil the syrup for 10 minutes. Take the pan from the heat and wait until the syrup stops bubbling. Pour in the brandy.

Pour the hot cordial into hot, sterilised bottles and cork it tightly. Fills about 1½ wine bottles.

Elderberry and Apple Pie

If you only have a few elderberries, add them to apples to make a pie.

pastry:
250 g (9 oz) wholewheat flour
pinch sea salt
175 g (6 oz) butter
60 ml (4 tablespoons) water
beaten egg for glaze
filling:
125 g (4 oz) elderberries, weighed on stem
450 g (1 lb) cooking apples
150 ml (¼ pint) dry cider
125 g (4 oz) honey
30 ml (2 tablespoons) tapioca or sago

Make the pastry and leave it in a cool place. Remove the elderberries from the stems. Peel, core and thinly slice the apples. Put the cider and honey into a saucepan. Set them on a low heat and stir until the honey dissolves. Bring them to the boil and add the apple slices. Cook them gently for

5 minutes. Take the pan from the heat and mix in the elderberries and tapioca or sago. Leave the fruits until they are cold.

Heat the oven to Reg 6/200C/400F. Roll out two thirds of the pastry and use it to line an 18 cm (7 inch) diameter 5 cm (2 inch) deep pie plate. Put in the apples and elderberries and all the juices. Cover them with the remaining pastry. Seal the edges and brush the top with beaten egg.

Bake the pie for 30 minutes or until it is golden brown. Serve it hot with single or soured cream. Serves 4.

To make wine taste as though it is made of Muscat Grapes

Open a bottle of good white wine. Pour a little off and drink it. Push one large head of elderflowers into the bottle and replace the cork. Leave the wine at room temperature for 24 hours. Remove the elderflower sprig and chill the wine very slightly before serving.

You can flavour natural apple juice or sweet cider in the same way.

Elderflower Champagne

Elderflower champagne is pale coloured and sparkling and very refreshing. It is made using a slightly different method from that of other wines.

Do make sure the bottles are proper champagne bottles and that the corks are securely wired on.

850 ml (1½ pints) elderflowers
2 oranges, rind and pith removed
juice 1 lemon
4.6 litres (1 gallon) water
1.35 kg (3 lbs) sugar
champagne yeast
yeast nutrient
250 ml (8 fl oz) strong cold black tea
450 g (1 lb) raisins, chopped

Pick the elderflowers when they are fully open and the pollen is dusty. Hold the sprigs over a container and hit them against a wooden spoon so the flowers fall off. Discard the sprigs. To the flowers add the sliced oranges and the lemon juice. Pour on 2.3 litres (4 pints) boiling water. Cover, then leave in a warm place for 10 days.

Make a syrup with the sugar and 2.3 litres (4 pints) boiling water. Put it into a container and strain on the elderflower liquid. Leave until luke-warm. Add the yeast, yeast nutrient and tea. Put the mixture into a 4.6 litre (1 gallon) jar and add the raisins. Fit a fermentation lock and leave for three weeks at a temperature of 21–24C (70–75F). Rack the liquid into champagne bottles adding 2.5 ml (½ teaspoon) sugar to each bottle. Wire or tie on the corks.

Leave the champagne for at least three months before opening.

Elderberry and Apple Wine

Elderberries and apples make a light red wine. If you have enough crab apples, you can use those instead of cultivated apples.

1.35 kg (3 lbs) elderberries, weighed on stems
2.7 kg (4 lbs) apples
4.6 litres (1 gallon) water
juice 4 lemons
Burgundy yeast
yeast nutrient
pectolase
1.35 kg (3 lbs) sugar

String the elderberries. Put them into a container and crush them. Wash, chop and pulp the apples.

Put the apples into a pan with the water. Bring them to the boil and boil them for 15 minutes. Strain the liquid onto the elderberries. Cool the mixture to lukewarm and add the yeast, yeast nutrient and pectolase.

Cover the brew and leave it in a warm place to fement for four to five days, stirring every day.

Strain the liquid onto a syrup made with the sugar and 575 ml (1 pint) water. Pour it into a 4.6 litre (1 gallon) jar and fit a fermentation lock. Rack as the wine clears and bottle when fermentation is complete.

Leave the wine for at least a year before opening. If possible, leave it for three years, as the older elderberry wine is the better.

Cosmetic

To whiten and soften the skin: Sew dried elder flowers into a muslin bag and steep it in the bath water. This is also said to have a very calming effect.

To tone and cleanse the face: Infuse 50 g (2 oz) elderflower sprigs in 575 ml (1 pint) boiling water for 24 hours. Strain and add the juice of 1 lemon and 150 ml (¼ pint) eau de cologne. Bottle and use as a face wash every morning.

Medicinal

A spring blood purifier: Infuse 1 sprig fresh elderflowers in 275 ml (½ pint) boiling water for 10 minutes. Strain. Drink the whole amount every morning before breakfast for three weeks.

For headaches: Make the above infusion. Cool it completely. Soak a cloth in it and lie down with a cloth over your forehead.

An ointment for sprains and chilblains

225 g (8 oz) young elder leaves, bruised
175 g (6 oz) petroleum jelly
25 g (1 oz) beeswax

Put the petroleum jelly and beeswax into a small, flameproof casserole and melt them together on a low heat without letting them boil. Stir in the elder leaves. Cover the casserole and put it into a low oven (Reg under ¼/70C/200F) for 4 hours. Working quickly, before the ointment has a chance to set, strain it through muslin or a nylon sieve into a jar. Let it cool and firm and cover it.

For chapped hands and chilblains: Make an ointment with 125 g (4 oz) elderflower sprigs in the same way as the elder leaf ointment.

To keep eyes strong and healthy: Infuse 10 ml (2 teaspoons) chopped elder leaves in 575 ml (1 pint) boiling water until cold. Strain. Use this infusion regularly to bathe the eyes.

Cold remedies: Infuse 15 g (½ oz) dried elder flowers in 275 ml (½ pint) boiling water for 10 minutes. Strain, sweeten with honey and drink the whole amount, hot on going to bed.
Infuse 7.5 ml (½ tablespoon) each dried elderflowers, yarrow and peppermint leaves in 275 ml (½ pint) boiling water for 10 minutes. Strain and sweeten with honey. Drink the whole amount, hot, on going to bed and take the same infusion three times during the following day and again at bed time.
Boil 125 g (4 oz) fresh or 50 g (2 oz) dried berries in 575 ml (1 pint) water for 15 minutes. Strain and sweeten with honey. Drink half the amount, hot, twice a day.
Drink hot elderberry wine or elderberry rob on going to bed early.

Influenza remedies: Infuse 15 g (½ oz) each dried elderflowers and peppermint leaves in 575 ml (1 pint) water for ½ hour. Strain and sweeten with honey. Reheat and drink in cupfuls, as hot as possible, whilst in bed.
Put 15 g (½ oz) dried elderflowers and 25 g (1 oz) dried peppermint leaves into a saucepan with 575 ml (1 pint) boiling water. Simmer for 15–20 minutes. Strain, sweeten and drink half the amount, hot, on going to bed and the rest first thing the following morning.

To prevent insect bites: Wear bruised elder leaves in your hair.
Infuse 25 g (1 oz) chopped elder leaves in 575 ml (1 pint) boiling water until cool. Use the infusion to wash over your face, hands and arms before gardening.

Veterinary

To keep gad-fly away from cattle and horses, boil four handfuls of green stalks and leaves of elder in 2.3 litres (4 pints) water. Leave until cool and use as a wash.
For wounds and skin disorders, boil two handfuls elder blossoms or chopped leaves in 850 ml (1½ pints) water for 5 minutes. Leave until cold and strain. Use to bathe the affected part.

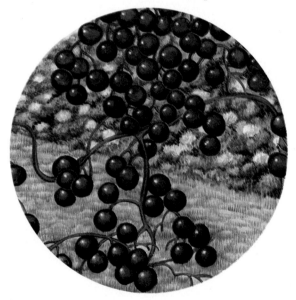

FIELD MUSHROOM

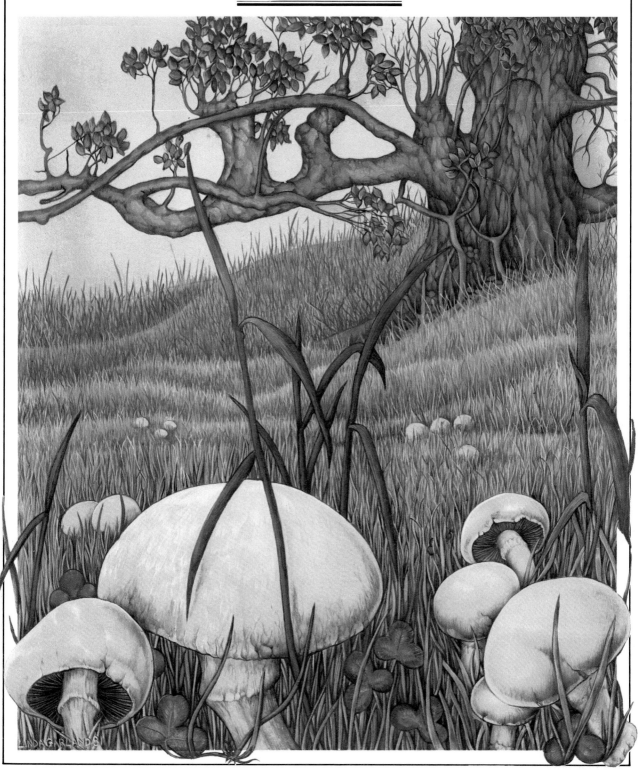

Availability

The field mushroom grows throughout Britain, Scandinavia, Europe, North America and Australia. It is to be found mainly on rich pasture-land and in established orchards, particularly where animals have been grazing. If you are lucky, you may sometimes find them growing on your lawn. When the weather has been dry they also grow on dung heaps.

The main season for field mushrooms is from late August to October (February to April in Australasia). They can be picked at all times of the day, but many people prefer the early morning.

For the sake of safe identification, leave field mushrooms when they are only at the button stage and wait until they are cup-shaped or fully open. Do not eat any mushrooms that are not positively identified.

If you pull a mushroom from the ground by hand, always make sure that you cut off the end of the stipe (stalk) with a sharp knife on the spot, letting the unwanted piece fall to the ground. It is believed that this will help the mushroom re-propagate. You can also gather mushrooms by cutting them at the base of the stipe.

You do not need to peel field mushrooms but always cut them open before cooking to make sure that they are free from maggots.

Mushroom and Avocado Soup

225 g (8 oz) field mushrooms, at the cup stage
25 g (1 oz) butter
1 large onion, finely chopped
15 ml (1 tablespoon) flour
850 ml (1½ pints) stock
bouquet garni
2 ripe avocados
30 ml (2 tablespoons) chopped parsley

Finely chop the mushrooms. Melt the butter in a saucepan on a low heat. Stir in the mushrooms and the onion. Cover them and cook them gently for 10 minutes. Stir in the flour and cook it for ½ minute. Stir in the stock and bring it to the boil. Add the bouquet garni and simmer, uncovered, for 15 minutes.

Peel, stone and dice the avocados. Remove the bouquet garni and put the soup into a blender with the avocados. Work it until it is thick and smooth. Reheat the soup if necessary and serve it garnished with the parsley. Serves 4.

Aubergine (Eggplant) and Mushroom Kebabs

Serve this as a first course.

1 large aubergine (eggplant) weighing 350–450 g (12 oz–1 lb)
15 ml (1 tablespoon) sea salt
225 g (8 oz) open field mushrooms
90 mll (6 tablespoons) olive oil
juice 1 lemon
freshly ground black pepper
sauce:
275 ml (½ pint) natural yoghurt
30 ml (2 tablespoons) tomato purée

5 ml (1 teaspoon) ground paprika
5 ml (1 teaspoon) ground cinnamon
1 clove garlic, crushed with a pinch sea salt

Cut the aubergine (eggplant) into 2 cm (¾ inch) dice. Put them into a collander and sprinkle them with the salt. Leave them to drain for 30 minutes. Rinse them under cold water and pat them dry with kitchen paper. Halve or quarter the mushrooms, depending on their size. Beat the oil, lemon juice and pepper together in a bowl and fold in the aubergines and mushrooms. Leave them for at least 2 hours at room temperature.

To make the sauce, beat the yoghurt with the rest of the ingredients. When you are ready to cook, alternate pieces of aubergine and mushroom on kebab skewers. Heat the grill/broiler to high. Lay the kebabs on the hot rack and grill/broil them for 10 minutes, turning them several times. Serve the kebabs on individual plates with the sauce spooned over them. Serves 4.

Mushroom Tart

shortcrust pastry made with 225 g (8 oz) wholewheat flour
225 g (8 oz) field mushrooms
40 g (1½ oz) butter
2 medium onions, halved and thinly sliced
30 ml (2 tablespoons) chopped thyme
10 ml (2 teaspoons) chopped rosemary
15 ml (1 tablespoon) chopped savory
75 g (3 oz) Cheddar cheese
5 eggs
sea salt and freshly ground black pepper

Heat the oven to Reg 6/200C/400F. Make the

pastry and chill it. Melt the butter in a frying pan on a low heat. Mix in the onions and cook them until they are soft. Raise the heat, put in the mushrooms and stir them about for ½ minute. Take the pan from the heat and mix in the herbs. Cool the contents slightly. Roll out the pastry and use it to line a 25 cm (10 inch) diameter flan tin. Put the mushroom mixture in the bottom. Finely grate the cheese and scatter it over the mushrooms. Beat the eggs with the seasonings and pour them over the cheese, moving them about with a fork to make sure they are evenly distributed. Bake the tart for 30 minutes so the top goes a good golden brown. Serves 6.

Lemon and Mushroom Stuffing for Chicken

This is good if you only manage to find a few mushrooms. It makes sure everyone gets a share. The amount will fill an average sized roasting chicken.

125 g (4 oz) field mushrooms
25 g (1 oz) butter
1 medium onion, finely chopped
100 g (3½ oz) wholewheat breadcrumbs
15 ml (1 tablespoon) chopped parsley
15 ml (1 tablespoon) chopped lemon thyme
grated rind half lemon and juice of 1 lemon
sea salt and freshly ground black pepper

Finely chop the mushrooms. Melt the butter in a frying pan on a low heat. Mix in the onion and cook it until it is soft. Raise the heat to moderate, put in the mushrooms and cook them for 2 minutes, stirring them around frequently. Take the pan from the heat and mix in the breadcrumbs, herbs and lemon rind. Bind everything together with the lemon juice and season lightly. Let the stuffing cool before you put it into the chicken.

Braised Brisket and Mushrooms in Beer

1 piece lean rolled brisket weighing around 1 kg
    (2–2½ lbs)
15 g (½ oz) beef dripping
1 medium onion, thinly sliced
1 clove garlic, finely chopped
275 ml (½ pint) bitter beer
15 ml (1 tablespoon) tomato purée
30 ml (2 tablespoons) chopped parsley
15 ml (1 tablespoon) chopped thyme
350 g (12 oz) field mushrooms, cut into 2.5 cm (1 inch)
    pieces

Heat the oven to Reg 4/180C/350F. Melt the

dripping in a large flameproof casserole on a high heat. Put in the beef and brown it all over. Remove it, lower the heat, stir in the onion and garlic and cook them until they are soft. If there is any excess fat in the pan at this point, pour or spoon it away. Pour in the beer and bring it to the boil. Stir in the tomato purée, parsley and thyme. Replace the beef and surround it with the mushrooms. Cover the casserole and put it into the oven for 1½ hours. Take out the beef, carve it and arrange it on a serving dish. Skim the juices in the pan if necessary and spoon them and the mushrooms over the beef. Serve with horseradish sauce. Serves 4.

Stuffed Field Mushrooms

When you find really large field mushrooms it is worthwhile stuffing them and using them as a base for a main dish. Although these mushrooms are used whole, slit them part way through before cooking just to check that they are sound and then press them together again.

8 large, flat field mushrooms, each about 10–12 cm (4–5
    inches) diameter
50 g (2 oz) butter
1 medium onion, finely chopped
125 g (1 cup) wholewheat breadcrumbs
125 g (4 oz) Cheshire or Cheddar cheese, grated
60 ml (4 tablespoons) chopped chives
8 sage leaves, chopped
125 ml (4 fl oz) dry cider

Heat the oven to Reg 6/200C/400F. Remove the stalks from the mushrooms and chop them. Melt the butter in a frying pan on a low heat. Take the pan from the heat and use half the butter to brush both sides of the mushrooms. Put the mushrooms, dark side up, in a flat, ovenproof dish. Soften the onion in the remaining butter and then mix in the mushroom stalks. Take the pan from the heat and mix in the rest of the ingredients. Pile the mixture on top of the mushrooms. Bake the mushrooms for 15 minutes. Serves 4.

HAZEL

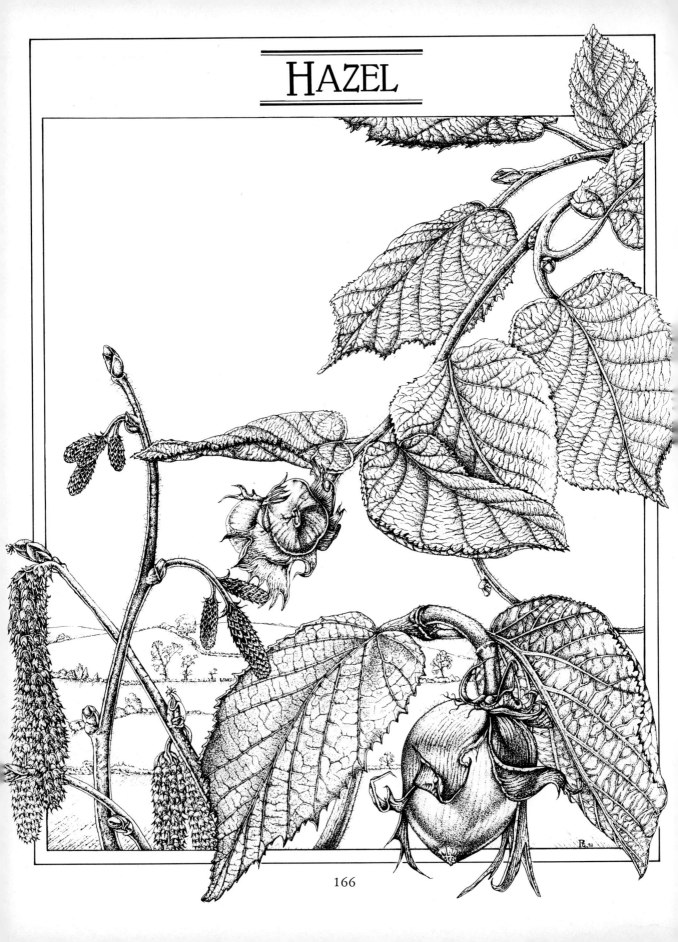

Availability

Hazel trees grow throughout Britain, Scandinavia and Europe, and can be found in woodland, in hedgerows and on scrub land. In the United States there are two related species. The American hazelnut (Corylus americana) can be found in the eastern, mid-western, southern and plains states; and the beaked hazelnut (Corylus rostrata) mainly in the mid-western and southern states. A variety of the beaked hazelnut also grows in California.

Hazelnuts become ready for picking in late summer and can be gathered until early autumn (August to October in the northern hemisphere).

To Store Hazelnuts

Gather hazel nuts on a dry day, preferably at the end of a dry spell so the outer husks are dry. Lay them on sacking or on several layers of newspaper in a warm, sunny room for a few days, turning them frequently. After this, the husks should come off easily. Pack the nuts between layers of dry sand, sawdust or tightly screwed up newspaper. If possible, cover them with a tight lid to keep out the mice. Hazel nuts keep well for up to six months. With age, they will lose their initial fresh, milky texture and will become drier.

Shelling Hazel Nuts

Hazel nuts which weigh 225 g (8 oz) with their shells will weigh about 125 g (4 oz) after shelling. The recipes below give the unshelled weight.

Hazelnut and Cottage Cheese Salad

Hazelnuts and apples help to make plain cottage cheese into an attractive and tasty salad. Serve it as a light main meal.

225 g (8 oz) hazelnuts
400 g (1 lb) cottage cheese
pinch cayenne pepper
10 ml (2 teaspoons) ground paprika
2 crisp eating apples
2 sticks celery
50 g (2 oz) raisins

Shell the hazelnuts. Mix the cheese with the cayenne pepper and paprika. Core and finely chop the apples, reserving one apple quarter. Finely chop the celery.

Mix the hazelnuts, chopped apples, celery and raisins into the cheese. Put the salad into a serving dish. Cut the reserved apple quarter into four thin lengthways slices and arrange them in a star on the top. Serves 4.

Hazel and Kiwi Fruit Salad

This makes an attractive and refreshing first course.

350 g (12 oz) hazel nuts
225 g (8 oz) cream cheese
pinch cayenne pepper
4 kiwi fruits

Shell the hazel nuts and finely chop all but 20 of them. Mix the chopped nuts into the cream cheese. Season with the cayenne pepper.

Skin the kiwi fruits and cut each one into five slices. Arrange the slices on each of four small plates, one in the centre and the rest round the edge.

Put a portion of the hazelnut cheese on each slice of kiwi fruit and top it with a whole nut. Serves 4.

Hazelnut Cake

This rich cake is absolutely packed with nuts, which keep their crisp, milky texture. If you haven't enough hazelnuts, a mixture of hazelnuts and walnuts or even unroasted peanuts can be used, giving a shelled weight of around 225 (8 oz).

450 g (1 lb) hazelnuts
175 g (6 oz) butter
125 g (4 oz) light brown (Barbados) sugar
125 g (4 oz) wholewheat flour
2.5 ml (½ teaspoon) ground cinnamon
2 eggs, beaten

Heat the oven to Reg 4/180C/350F. Shell and finely chop the hazelnuts. Melt the butter on a low heat. Stir in the sugar and cool them slightly.

Put the flour and cinnamon into a bowl. Make a well in the centre and pour in the butter and sugar. Add the eggs. Stir in the hazelnuts and mix well.

Pour the mixture into a buttered and floured 18 cm (7 inch) square cake tin. Bake the cake for 30 minutes so it is golden brown and has shrunk slightly from the sides of the tin. Cool the cake in the tin for 5 minutes and turn it onto a wire rack to cool completely.

Spaghetti with Hazelnuts and a thick Cheese Sauce

With a salad or a green vegetable, this rich spaghetti dish is a meal in itself

225 g (8 oz) wholewheat spaghetti
225 g (8 oz) hazelnuts
60 g (2½ oz) butter
1 clove garlic, crushed with a pinch sea salt
15 ml (1 tablespoon) chopped thyme
30 ml (2 tablespoons) chopped parsley
freshly ground black pepper
45 ml (3 tablespoons) flour
425 ml (¾ pint) milk
250 g (9 oz) Cheddar cheese, grated
sea salt

Boil the spaghetti in lightly salted water until it is just tender. Drain it in a collander and run cold water through it.

Shell the hazelnuts and grind them in a blender or clean coffee grinder. Melt 25 g (1 oz) of the butter in a saucepan. Stir in the garlic and cook it until it just begins to brown. Stir in the herbs and hazelnuts. Fold in the spaghetti, making sure that it gets well coated with the nut mixture. Season liberally with pepper and keep it warm.

In another saucepan, melt the remaining butter on a medium heat. Stir in the flour and cook it for 1 minute. Pour in the milk and bring it to the boil, stirring. Simmer the sauce for 2 minutes and take it from the heat. Beat in all the cheese.

Divide the spaghetti between four plates and spoon the cheese sauce over the top. Serves 4.

Hazelnut and Cauliflower Bake

This is like a savoury, light textured, baked omelette. Serve it as a main course.

225 g (8 oz) hazelnuts
1 small cauliflower
1 small onion
150 ml (¼ pint) stock
bouquet garni
4 eggs
75 g (3 oz) Cheddar cheese, grated
15 ml (1 tablespoon) tomato purée
30 ml (2 tablespoons) chopped parsley
10 ml (2 teaspoons) chopped marjoram
butter for greasing

Heat the oven to Reg 6/200C/400F. Shell the hazelnuts and grind them in a blender or clean coffee grinder. Cut the cauliflower into small fleurettes and thinly slice the onion.

Bring the stock to the boil in a saucepan. Put in the cauliflower, onion and bouquet garni. Cover and cook on a moderate heat for 10 minutes so the cauliflower is just tender and most of the stock evaporated. Remove the bouquet garni and either mash the cauliflower and onion with a potato masher or put them through the fine blade of a vegetable mill.

Beat the eggs and mix in the cheese, tomato purée and herbs. Mix in the cauliflower purée and ground hazelnuts. Pour the mixture into a buttered, 23 cm (9 inch) diameter 5 cm (2 inch) deep oven proof dish and bake it for 30 minutes so it is golden brown and risen. Serves 4.

Apple Mousse and Hazelnut Tart

Ground hazelnuts, muesli base and honey make a light textured sweet shell for a creamy mousse of apples and honey.

450 g (1 lb) hazelnuts
65 g (2½ oz) butter
125 g (4 oz) honey
5 ml (1 teaspoon) ground cinnamon
275 g (10 oz) muesli base
filling:
450 g (1 lb) cooking apples
45 ml (3 tablespoons) honey
120 ml (6 tablespoons) dry cider (or water)
5 ml (1 teaspoon) ground cinnamon
15 g (½ oz) gelatin
2 eggs, separated
150 ml (¼ pint) thick cream

Shell the hazelnuts. Toast them in a moderate oven for 10 minutes, cool them a little and rub off the skins. Reserve thirteen of them. Grind the rest in a blender or clean coffee grinder.

Put 50 g (2 oz) of the butter with the honey and cinnamon into a saucepan and set them on a low heat for the butter and honey to melt. Stir in the nuts and the muesli base and keep stirring until the muesli base becomes quite soaked in the butter mixture.

Use the remaining butter to grease a 25 cm (10 inch) diameter flan tin. Press the muesli mixture over the base and sides of the tin in an even layer. Put this shell into the refrigerator to set into shape while you make the filling.

Peel, core and chop the apples. Put them into a saucepan with the honey and 60 ml (4 tablespoons) of the cider. Add the cinnamon. Cover them and set them on a low heat for about 15 minutes, so they can be beaten to a purée. Rub them through a sieve.

Soak the gelatin in the remaining cider. Return the apple purée to the saucepan and set it on a low heat. Beat in the egg yolks and stir, without boiling, until the mixture will coat the back of a wooden spoon. Melt the gelatin in a small pan and stir it into the apple mixture. Take the pan from the heat and cool the apples until they are on the point of setting.

Whip the cream until it is thick and stiffly whip the egg whites. Fold half the cream into the apples and then all the whites. Pour the mousse mixture into the refrigerated shell and chill it for about an hour for it to set.

Put a small portion of whipped cream in the centre of the tart and twelve more round the edge. Top each one with a hazelnut. Serves 6.

Buttered Hazelnut Tart

The filling for this tart has a smooth, buttery consistency and a honeyed flavour.

shortcrust pastry made with 225 ml (8 oz) wholewheat
  flour
225 g (8 oz) hazelnuts
50 g (2 oz) light brown (Barbados) sugar
3 eggs, lightly beaten
175 g (6 oz) honey
juice ½ lemon
2 egg whites, stiffly beaten

Heat the oven to Reg 8/230C/450F. Line a 25 cm (10 inch) diameter tart tin with the pastry. Shell and finely chop the hazelnuts.

Use an electric beater to make the filling. Beat the butter and sugar together and gradually add the beaten egg. Add the honey and lemon juice and keep beating so the mixture becomes slightly frothy. Fold in first the chopped hazelnuts and then the egg whites.

Pour the mixture into the pastry case. Bake the tart for 10 minutes. Reduce the heat to Reg 4/180C/350F and bake for a further 25 minutes. The filling should be very brown on top and completely set. Let the tart get cold before serving. Serves 6.

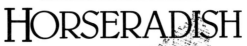
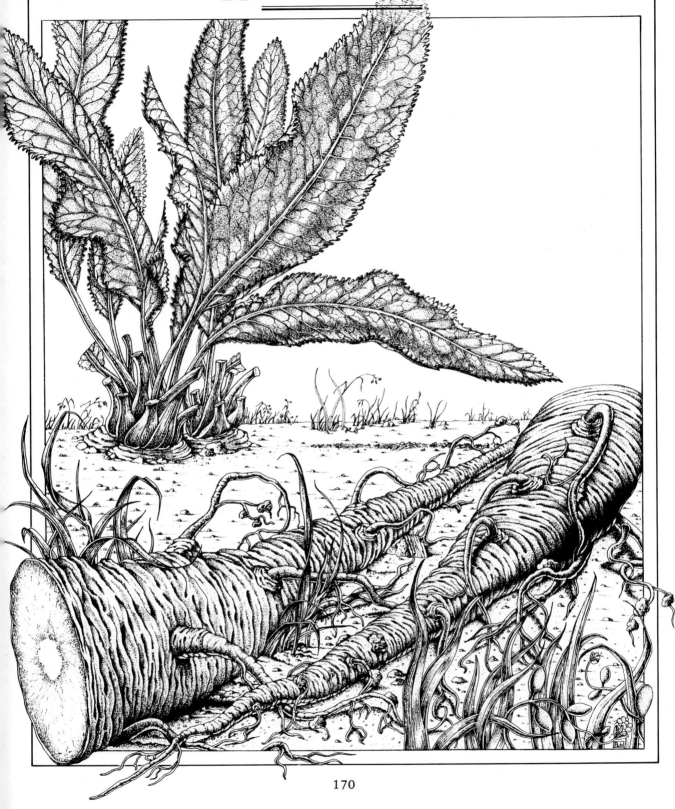

Availability

Horseradish can be found throughout the southern parts of Britain and Europe. It was introduced to the United States by European immigrants and grown originally as a garden plant. It can now be found growing wild mainly in the eastern states.

Horseradish grows on waste ground, on the sites of abandoned gardens and on railway banks. It thrives on moist ground and can often be found growing beside brooks.

The roots of horseradish should be dug in the autumn after the first frost (October and November in the northern hemisphere). Dig deep, using a large spade for they are very long and irregularly shaped. The roots will keep fresh for up to three days in a cool, dark place.

To Preserve Horseradish

Scrub the roots well but do not peel them unless they are very knobbly or blemished. Cut away any soft pieces.

Now get yourself prepared because working with horseradish, although worth it in the end, is one of the most unpleasant jobs in the countryside cook's year. Use either a surgeon's or a welder's mask or tie a cotton scarf round your face, cow-boy style, and line it with several layers of paper towels. If you have extra-sensitive eyes, swimmers' goggles may also help! It looks quite ridiculous but horseradish makes both eyes and nose run and it is quite unpleasant to breath in the fumes from large quantities of the freshly grated root.

If you only have a small amount of horseradish (up to 450 g (1 lb)) then it is possible to use a fine hand grater. If you have more then you should definitely use a robust blender or food processor. Work the horseradish until it is finely grated.

Keeping as far away from the appliance as possible, quickly remove the lid and turn the horseradish into a bowl. Cover it while you prepare the next batch.

Pack the horseradish fairly tightly into jars and then pour in white wine vinegar. Cover the horseradish and leave it for about 15 minutes for the vinegar to settle. Pour in more vinegar, cover and wait again. The horseradish should be just covered with the vinegar. You may have to pour in the vinegar in three or four stages depending on how tightly you have packed the horseradish. About 275 ml (½ pint) vinegar is needed per 450 g (1 lb) horseradish.

Seal the jars with plastic tops and store the horseradish in a cool, dark place. It should keep for up to six months.

Horseradish Sauce

This is a good, basic recipe for horseradish sauce. The soured cream gives a lighter flavour than whipped cream.

175 g (3 oz) horseradish
5 ml (1 teaspoon) dried mustard powder
10 ml (2 teaspoons) white wine or cider vinegar
150 ml (¼ pint) soured cream

Put the horseradish into a bowl and scatter in the mustard powder. Mix in the vinegar and soured cream. Leave the sauce for 15 minutes before serving.

The sauce will keep for up to two weeks in a covered container in the refrigerator.

Horseradish and Tomato Sauce

Add 30 ml (2 tablespoons) tomato purée and the grated rind of half a medium orange to the basic sauce. Good with mackerel, smoked mackerel and trout.

Horseradish, Orange and Tomato Relish

Serve this relish hot with sausages or with grilled fresh or smoked mackerel.

225 g (8 oz) tomatoes
1 small onion
30 ml (2 tablespoons) grated horseradish
grated rind and juice 1 large orange
10 ml (2 teaspoons) ground paprika
1.5 ml (¼ teaspoon) cayenne pepper
30 ml (2 tablespoons) white wine vinegar

Scald, skin and finely chop the tomatoes. Finely chop the onion. Put these with all the rest of the ingredients into a saucepan. Set them on a low heat and bring them to the boil. Simmer gently, uncovered, for 45 minutes so you have a thick relish.

Apple and Horseradish Sauce

Serve this with herrings and mackerel and cold salt beef.

2 medium sized cooking apples
30 ml (2 tablespoons) water
30 ml (2 tablespoons) soured cream
30 ml (2 tablespoons) grated horseradish

Peel, core and chop the apples. Put them into a saucepan with the water. Cover them and set them on a low heat for 15 minutes so you can beat them to a purée.

Take the pan from the heat and beat in the soured cream and horseradish. Put the sauce into a bowl and let it cool completely.

Sweet Horseradish and Beetroot Relish

This bright coloured sweet and sour relish goes superbly with cold beef, all cheese dishes, quiches and bread and cheese. Eat it immediately or keep it for up to a week in a covered container in the refrigerator.

125 g (4 oz) cooked beetroot
½ small cooking apple
50 g (2 oz) raisins
45 ml (3 tablespoons) grated horseradish
60 ml (4 tablespoons) red wine vinegar

Finely grate the beetroot and peel, core and finely chop the apple. Finely chop the raisins. Mix them all in a bowl with the horseradish and vinegar.

Beef in its own Horseradish Sauce

Beef and horseradish are the classic combination whether served separately or cooked together.

675–900 g (1½–2 lbs) beef skirt
275 ml (½ pint) stock
1 large onion, thinly sliced
30 ml (2 tablespoons) grated horseradish
30 ml (2 tablespoons) malt vinegar
60 ml (4 tablespoons) chopped parsley

Trim any fat and skin from the meat. Cut the meat into eight even sized pieces.

Put the stock into a heavy saucepan with the onion, horseradish and vinegar and bring it to the boil. Put in the beef and turn it quickly to sear both sides. Put the parsley on top, cover and simmer for 1 hour.

Most of the stock should boil down, leaving a fairly thick horseradish and onion sauce. Serve it spooned over the beef.

Smoked Mackerel and Horseradish Pâté

Horseradish and mackerel go together superbly, whether served separately or mixed to make a pâté.

2 smoked whole mackerel, each weighing about 225 g (8 oz)
75 ml (2 tablespoons) grated horseradish
15 ml (1 tablespoon) white wine vinegar
grated rind and juice ½ medium orange
45 ml (3 tablespoons) chopped parsley

Slit open the mackerel and remove all the bones. Put the flesh and any roes into a large basin and pound them to a paste. Work in the soured cream, horseradish, vinegar, orange rind and juice and parsley.

Press the pâté into a small dish or terrine and chill it until it is firm, about 1 hour.

Serves 6 as a first course, 3–4 as a main course.

Horseradish and Pickled Onion Sauce

Add three very finely chopped pickled onions to the basic sauce. This is good with cold beef.

Minced Beef, Mushrooms and Horseradish

675 g (1½ lbs) minced or ground beef
1 large onion, thinly sliced
225 g (8 oz) mushrooms, thinly sliced
60 ml (4 tablespoons) chopped parsley
200 ml (7 fl oz) barley wine (or other very strong beer)
30 ml (2 tablespoons) grated horseradish
30 ml (2 tablespoons) malt vinegar

Heat a large sauté pan or flameproof casserole on a high heat without any fat. Put in the meat and break it up well. Stir it about until it browns.

Put in the onion and mushrooms and keep stirring on the heat for about 2 minutes so the onion begins to soften. Add the parsley and pour in the barley wine. Bring it to the boil. Cover the pan tightly and keep it on a very low heat for 30 minutes.

Soak the horseradish in the vinegar. Stir it into the beef, cover again and cook for a further 2 minutes. Serves 4.

Veal with Mustard, Capers, Horseradish and Lemon

Serve this light veal dish with wholemeal pasta.

675 g (1½ lbs) pie veal
25 g (1 oz) butter
225 g (8 oz) mushrooms
10 ml (2 teaspoons) dried mustard powder
15 ml (1 tablespoon) grated horseradish
30 ml (2 tablespoons) chopped capers
juice 1 lemon
10 ml (6 tablespoons) stock

Cut the veal into 1.5 cm (½ inch) cubes. Thinly slice the mushrooms. Heat the butter in a heavy sauté pan or wide based casserole on a high heat. Put in the veal and brown it. Put in the mushrooms and stir for 1 minute.

Turn the heat to the lowest point. Stir in the mustard, capers, horseradish, lemon juice and stock. Cover the pan and keep it on a very low heat for 25 minutes. Serves 4.

Horseradish and Chilli Vinegar

Use this vinegar for making mayonnaise and salad dressing and for sauces for fish.

one 375 ml (13 fl oz) bottle white wine vinegar
30 ml (2 tablespoons) grated horseradish
2 dried red chillies

Pour off and set aside about 90 ml (6 tablespoons) vinegar. Put the horseradish and chillies into the bottle and top up with as much of the reserved vinegar as will go back into the bottle.

Leave the bottle on a sunny windowsill for 3 weeks.

Cosmetic

To produce a clear, fresh skin: Steep 30 ml (2 tablespoons) freshly grated horseradish in 275 ml (½ pint) milk for 4 hours. Strain and use as a lotion.

Medicinal

To aid digestion: Eat horseradish with oily fish and rich meats.

To relieve chilblains: Cover them with grated fresh horseradish root and secure it with a bandage.

To relieve a heavy head cold: Inhale the fumes of freshly grated horseradish.

To relieve the cough that follows influenza: Eat horseradish regularly with meals.

Veterinary

Horseradish is a warming plant and a little grated root can be added to the horses' feed during the winter.

To stimulate the appetite and as a general tonic, steep 10 ml (2 teaspoons) grated horseradish root in 125 ml (4 fl oz) water for 4 hours. Strain and add to the feed.

For swellings, grate the fresh root and apply it to the affected part, securing it with a bandage.

ROWAN

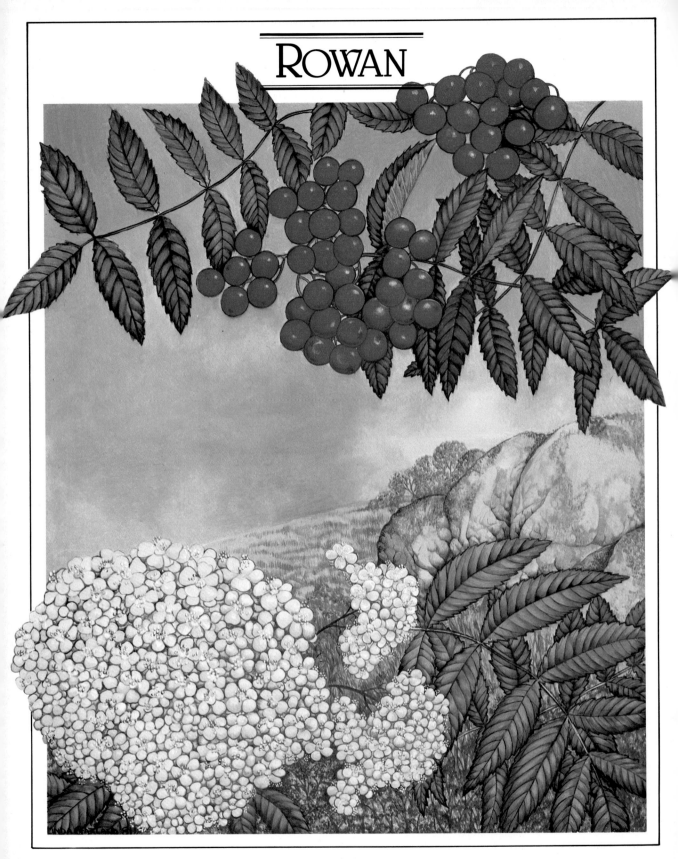

SORBUS AUCUPARIA

Local Names (Tree): Care, Care Tree, Chitchat, Quickbeam,
Quicken, Quicken-Tree, Quicken-Wood, Wicken,
Twickband, Twickbine, Whistle Tree, Wicky, Roddin,
Shepherd's Friend, Whistle Wood, Witchbeam, Witch Wood
(Berries): Cares, Cock-Drunks, Hen-Drunks, Dog Berries,
Poison Berries, Quicken Berries

Availability

The rowan tree grows throughout Britain but is more common in the north and north west. It can be found in most parts of Scandinavia and Europe.

In the wild, the rowan tree grows on heaths and moors and rocky uplands and in ancient woodland. It is also planted as a decorative tree along suburban roads and in parks and gardens.

In the United States the rowan is known as the European mountain ash. It is planted universally as a decorative tree and has established itself as an escape in some states. Two wild American species that can be used in the same ways are Sorbus americana and Sorbus scopulina.

The clusters of large, orange-red berries ripen from late summer to early autumn (August to October in the northern hemisphere). They are best left until after they have been softened by two frosts but you may have to pick them earlier for once they are ripe the birds will quickly eat them.

The clusters of berries can easily be broken off by hand. They will keep for several days in a cool place.

Spiced Roast Pork with Rowan Apples

Rowan jelly makes an attractive and tasty glaze for pork, and spooened over apples, a pretty garnish.

about 1.35 kg (3 lbs) thick end leg of pork
10 allspice berries
10 black peppercorns
5 ml (1 teaspoon) sea salt
1 large clove garlic
10 sage leaves
2 sprigs rosemary
3 small cooking apples
90 ml (6 tablespoons) rowan jelly
15 ml (1 tablespoon) wholewheat flour
275 ml (½ pint) stock
150 ml (¼ pint) dry cider

Heat the oven to Reg 4/180C/350F. Score the pork rind. Crush together the allspice berries, peppercorns and salt. Rub them all over the outside of the pork and well into the scores.

Cut very thin slivers of garlic. Chop the sage leaves into 65 mm (¼ inch) pieces and separate the rosemary leaves. Press these into the scores and down beside the bone as deep as possible. Separate the muscles of the meat and push garlic and herbs between them. Put the pork into a roasting tin and put it into the oven for 2 hours.

Peel and core the apples and cut them in half lengthways. Put the halves, cut side down, round the pork and return the pork to the oven for 15 minutes. Spoon 7.5 ml (½ tablespoon) rowan jelly over each apple half and 30 ml (2 tablespoons) over the pork. Return the pork to the oven for a further 5 minutes.

Take out the pork and put it onto a carving plate. Surround it with the apples and keep it warm. Pour any excess fat from the pan and set the pan on top of the stove on a moderate heat. Stir in the flour and cook it for ½ minute. Pour in the stock and cider and bring them to the boil, stirring in any residue from the bottom of the pan. Simmer the sauce for 2 minutes and serve it separately. Serves 6.

Rowan Jelly

Rowan berries make a dark orange bitter-sweet jelly. Serve it with lamb, pork or game.

1.8 kg (4 lbs) rowan berries
900 g (2 lbs) crab apples or cooking apples
thinly pared rind and juice 1 lemon
5 cm (2 inch) piece cinnamon stick
5 ml (1 teaspoon) cloves
450 g (1 lb light brown (demerara) sugar
    to every 575 ml (1 pint) juice

Wash the rowan berries. Roughly chop the apples without peeling. Put the berries and apples into a preserving pan with the lemon rind and juice, cinnamon and cloves. Pour in water to just cover them. Bring them to the boil and simmer until the berries and apples are very soft, about 1 hour.

Turn the fruit into a jelly bag and let it drip. It will take quite a long time for all the juice to come through and you can leave the pulp in the bag to drip overnight.

Measure the juice and return it to the cleaned pan. Add the sugar and stir on a low heat for it to dissolve. Bring the juice to the boil and boil rapidly until setting point is reached.

Pour the jelly into warmed small pots and cover it with circles of waxed paper. Cover it completely when cold. Makes about 900 g (2 lbs).

Availability

The walnut is a native of the middle east which was brought very early to southern Europe. It now grows throughout Britain and Europe but is more common in southern areas. It can be found in old woodland, in parks and on the sites of abandoned gardens.

In the United States Juglans regia is called the English walnut and it is cultivated by grafting onto the black walnut. The black walnut (Juglans nigra) is the most widely spread walnut tree in the United States. It can be found in forests in the eastern, mid-western, plains and southern states and Texas. The small, thick shelled Texas walnut (Juglans rupestris) grows along canyons and streams of the south west; and the Californian walnut (Juglans californica) which is small, thin shelled and sweet tasting, grows all along the west coast.

Walnuts for pickling should be picked in summer (early and mid July in the northern hemisphere), when the shells are soft enough for you to be able to stick a thick needle right through them. Pickle them with the green husk still attached.

The nuts ripen in mid-autumn (late September and early October in the northern hemisphere). They should fall naturally from the trees so that all you have to do is come along and pick them up. Shaking branches or beating the tree will help obstinate nuts to drop.

If the leaves are required for medicinal purposes, gather them in mid-summer (June to July in the northern hemisphere) in fine weather. Dry them quickly so they retain their colour.

The bark, again for medicinal purposes, should be peeled off the tree in spring (April in the northern hemisphere) and dried.

To Prepare and Store Walnuts

When the nuts have been gathered in the autumn, the husks should be removed as soon as possible. Wear rubber gloves, otherwise your hand will be stained as brown as a gypsy's. Slit the husks all round with a small, sharp knife and gently prize them apart to leave the bare shells. Any pieces of husk still clinging to the shell should be scrubbed off as they have a tendency to go mouldy when the nuts are stored. Use a soft nailbrush and warm water.

After scrubbing, lay the nuts to dry on several layers of newspaper in a warm sunny room for about three days, turning them several times. Nuts used directly after this initial drying stage are known as "wet" walnuts and they will be crisp and milky textured. They are delicious to eat on their own and are very suitable for recipes which require them to be pounded.

As walnuts are stored, they become drier and more earthy flavoured, like those that can be bought around Christmas. If the summer has been a wet one, the shells of walnuts could very well be thin. If this is the case, use the nuts as soon as possible as they will dry and shrivel very quickly in the shell. Before storing, pick out any with cracked open shells and use them "wet".

The best way of storing walnuts is to layer them in a box with coconut fibre and salt, but not everyone has access to coconut fibre. Dry sawdust or tightly screwed up newspaper can be used instead, together with a liberal sprinkling of rock salt.

Shelling Walnuts

Twenty walnuts weighed in the shell produce about 125 g (4 oz) shelled nuts.

To Pickle Walnuts

This might seem rather a lengthy process of pickling, but it makes the nuts deliciously soft and spicy flavoured and is well worth the effort.

2.25 kg (5 lbs) green walnuts
1.425 kg (3 lb 6 oz) rock salt
15 ml (1 tablespoon) grated horseradish
6 shallots, sliced
2 cloves garlic per jar, peeled and left whole
2 litres (3½ pints) malt vinegar

Wash the walnuts. Put them into a large bowl and cover them with boiling water. Leave them until they are cool and a dull green colour. Dissolve 165 g (6 oz) salt in 1.7 litres (3 pints) cold water. Wearing rubber or polythene gloves, take the walnuts out of the water one by one and scrape off the thin outer skins. Drop them immediately into the brine. When they are all done, leave them for 24 hours.

Strain off the brine and once more pour boiling water over the walnuts. Make fresh brine with another 175 g (6 oz) salt and 1.7 litres (3 pints) water. Put in the walnuts and leave them for a further 24 hours. Do this every day for seven more days.

On the tenth day, pour off all the brine and cover the walnuts with cold water. Drain them. Layer them in jars with the mustard seeds, horse-radish and shallots, adding two peeled cloves of garlic to each jar, about one third and two thirds of the way up.

Put the vinegar into an enamelled or stainless steel pan and bring it to the boil. Cool it a little and pour it over the walnuts. Cover the jars tightly while they are still warm and leave them for two weeks before opening. They will keep for up to two years. Fills five 450 g (1 lb) jars.

Turkey Stuffed with Wild Apricots and Walnuts

This is a way of cooking turkey for special occasions. It is beautifully flavoured, looks superb and is very easy to carve. The stuffing is just as good cold as it is hot.

Wild apricots can be bought from wholefood shops. They are very dark in colour due to the fact that they have not been sulphured. If they are not available, use ordinary dried apricots.

one 4.5 kg (10 lb) turkey
75 g (3 oz) dried wild apricots
200 ml (7 fl oz) dry white wine
20 walnuts
25 g (1 oz) butter
1 large onion, finely chopped
175 g (6 oz) breadcrumbs
60 ml (4 tablespoons) chopped parsley

Soak the apricots overnight in the wine. Lay the turkey, breast down and slit it down the backbone. Follow the bone round with a sharp knife so you eventually remove the backbone and rib cage, but leave the leg and wing bones in place.

Heat the oven to Reg 4/180C/350F. Shell and finely chop the walnuts. Drain the apricots, reserving the wine, and finely chop them. Melt the butter in a frying pan on a low heat. Put in the onion and soften it. Take the pan from the heat and mix in the apricots, walnuts, breadcrumbs, parsley and the reserved liquid. Fill the turkey with the stuffing, reshape it and sew it up.

Put the turkey into a roasting tin and cover it completely with foil. Put it into the oven for 2 hours. Remove the foil and put the turkey back into the oven for a further hour so the skin crisps and becomes a deep brown. Serves 8–10.

Pumpkin and Walnut Pie

Pounded fresh walnuts add a nutty flavour and texture to a traditional pumpkin pie.

pastry:
225 g (8 oz) wholewheat flour
pinch sea salt
10 ml (2 teaspoons) baking powder
150 g (5 oz) butter or half butter and half white shortening
90 ml (6 tablespoons) cold water
filling:
20 wet walnuts
1.125 kg (2½ lbs) pumpkin, weighed before preparing
125 g (4 oz) honey
¼ nutmeg, grated
2.5 ml (½ teaspoon) ground cinnamon
2.5 ml (½ teaspoon) ground ginger
grated rind 1 lemon
grated rind ½ medium orange
4 eggs, beaten
150 ml (¼ pint) thick cream

Cut the rind from the pumpkin and leave it in a cool place. Heat the oven to Reg 4/180C/350F.

Cut the rind from the pumpkin and scoop out the seeds and pith. Cut the flesh into 4 cm (1½ inch) chunks and steam them for 15 minutes. Let them drain well. Put them into a bowl and mash them to a purée. Stir in the honey, spices and lemon and orange rinds. Leave the pumpkin until it is lukewarm.

Roll out the pastry and line a 20 cm (8 inch) diameter 5 cm (2 inch) deep flan ring. Shell the walnuts and roughly pound them.

Mix the walnuts, eggs and cream into the pumpkin. Bake the pie for 1 hour so the filling rises and browns on top. Serve it hot or cold. As the pie cools the filling will become flat again but it stays a delicious, creamy texture. Serves 6—8.

WALNUT

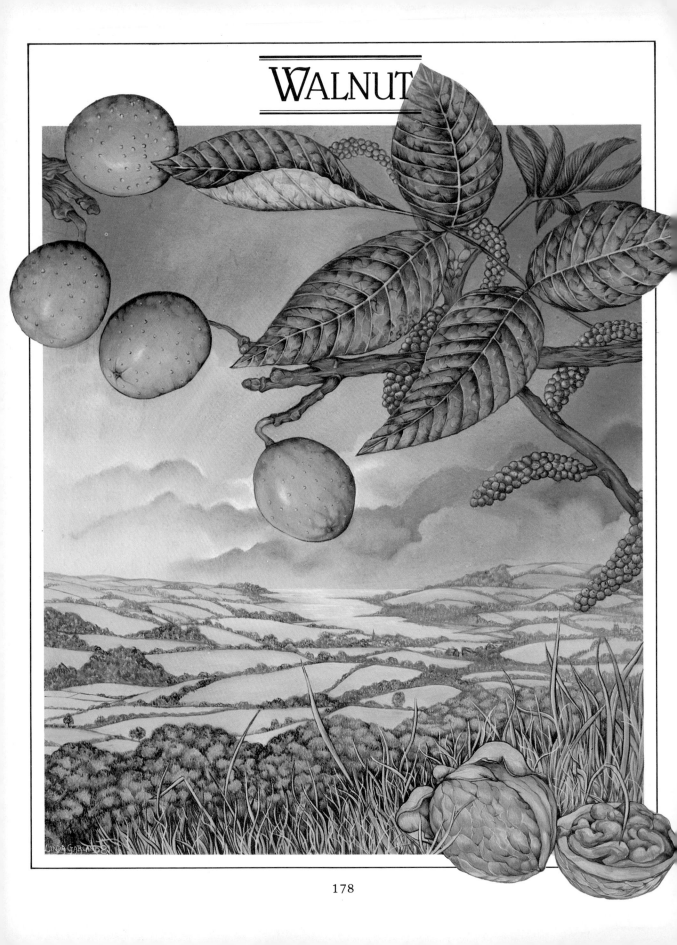

Brownie Cake

This is a fairly close textured but moist cake. Serve it plainly or decorate it with whipped cream and fresh fruits.

125 g (4 oz) plain carob chocolate
125 g (4 oz) butter
125 g (4 oz) light brown (Barbados) sugar
2 eggs, beaten
175 g (6 oz) wholewheat flour
15 walnuts, shelled and chopped

Heat the oven to Reg 4/180C/350F. Put the chocolate into a bowl. Stand the bowl in a saucepan of water and melt the chocolate on a low heat.

Beat the butter with the sugar until it is light and creamy. Beat in the chocolate. Beat in the eggs, alternately with the flour. Fold in the walnuts. Put the mixture into a buttered 20 cm (8 inch) diameter cake tin and bake it for 40 minutes or until a skewer inserted in the centre comes out clean.

Cool the cake in the tin for 5 minutes and turn it onto a wire rack to cool completely.

Veal, Pork and Walnut Terrine

Serve this terrine as a main meal, with a salad. It is very light in both texture and flavour.

450 g (1 lb) pie veal
450 g (1 lb) streaky pork rashers, rind and bones removed
20 wet walnuts, shelled
15 g (½ oz) pistachio nuts, (optional)
2.5 ml (½ teaspoon) ground mace
1.5 ml (¼ teaspoon) ground allspice
¼ nutmeg, grated
15 ml (1 tablespoon) mixed chopped thyme and marjoram
15 ml (1 tablespoon) chopped parsley
grated rind and juice of 1 small orange

Heat the oven to Reg 4/180C/350F. Mince the veal, pork and walnuts together. Cut the pistachio nuts (if using) in half. Mix them into the meats. Add the spices and herbs and mix well. Pack the mixture into a 900 g (2 lb) loaf tin. Cover it with foil.

Stand the tin in an oven tin of warm water. Put it into the oven for 1½ hours. Take it out of the oven tin. Press the terrine with a weight until it is quite cold. It is best left overnight. Turn it out of the loaf tin. Serve it cut into slices. Serves 4—6.

Walnut, Grapefruit and Kiwi Fruit Salad

Serve these attractive salads as a first course.

20 wet walnuts
1 clove garlic, finely chopped
2.5 ml (½ teaspoon) curry powder
90 ml (6 tablespoons) natural yoghurt
2 pink grapefruit
2 kiwi fruits

Shell the walnuts and reserve four of the best halves. Pound the rest to a paste, gradually adding the garlic, curry powder and yoghurt.

Peel the grapefruit. Cut them in half lengthways and then each half into five crossways slices. Peel the kiwi fruit and cut each one into six crossways slices.

Arrange five half slices of grapefruit in an overlapping line down the centre of each of four small plates. Put a portion of the walnut mixture in the centre. Put one slice of kiwi fruit on top and a reserved walnut half on top of that. Put another slice of kiwi fruit on either side of the line of grapefruit. Serves 4.

Avocados with Walnut Filling

Wet walnuts can be easily pounded to a creamy paste to make salad dressings. If walnut oil is too expensive, use sunflower oil.

2 ripe avocados
10 wet walnuts
1 clove garlic, finely chopped
30 ml (2 tablespoons) walnut oil
30 ml (2 tablespoons) white wine vinegar
freshly ground black pepper

Halve and stone the avocados. Shell the walnuts. Reserve four of the best halves and, using a large pestle and mortar, pound the rest to a paste adding the garlic when they begin to break up. Add the oil, wine vinegar and pepper and pound again to mix well.

Fill the centres of the avocados with the walnut mixture. Top them with the remaining walnut halves. Serves 4 as a first course, 2 as a main course.

Medicinal

For sore or ulcerated throats: Gargle with the vinegar in which green walnuts were pickled.

For skin troubles and eczema: Infuse 25 g (1 oz) dried walnut leaves or bark in 575 ml (1 pint) boiling water for 6 hours. Strain and take in wineglassful doses three times a day.
Or, put 10 ml (2 teaspoons) dried walnut leaves into a saucepan with 225 ml (8 fl oz) water and bring them to simmering point. Remove them from the heat and let stand for 5—10 minutes. Take the whole amount, twice a day, over several weeks.
Or, put 10 ml (2 teaspoons) dried leaves in 500 ml (16 fl oz) water and boil for 1 minute. Let the decoction stand for 20 minutes. Make a damp, loose compress with the cooled liquid and apply it for 1–2 hours, three times a day.

For chilblains, reddened hands and excessive perspiration of the hands and feet: Macerate 50 g (2 oz) dried walnut leaves in 1 litre (1¾ pints) water for 2 hours. Bring them gently to the boil and boil for 2 minutes. Leave to stand for 15 minutes. Strain and use the liquid to bathe the affected parts.

For luxuriant eyelashes and eyebrows: Moisten them morning and evening with the above decoction.

Veterinary

Fresh walnut leaves, mixed with litter in a kennel, will keep a dog free from fleas.
For skin parasites and ringworm: Put two handfuls of walnut leaves or six of the green husks into a saucepan with 1.15 litres (2 pints) water. Bring them to simmering point and keep them there for 3 minutes. Take them from the heat and leave them to stand for 6 hours. Strain and give one cupful three times a day.

Local names (Tree): Blackhaw, Buckthorn, Bullen, Bullison, Bullister, Egg-Pegg-Bush, Pig-in-the-Hedge, Srogg, Slaathorn, Slacenbush, Slon-Bush, Slon-Tree, Snag-Bush (Fruits): Bullens, Heg-Pegs, Hedge-Picks, Hedge Speaks, Slags, Snags, Winter Kecksies, Winter-Picks

Availability

The sloe can be found throughout Britain, Europe and Scandinavia, although it is less common in the extreme north. It grows in woods and along hedgerows.

The flowers usually appear before the leaves in early spring (March to April in the northern hemisphere). The small, dark, round fruits should be picked after the first frost (September to October in the northern hemisphere). The bushes have long spines so it is best to wear gloves when picking. Sloes will keep for up to four days in a cool place.

Sloes do not grow in the United States, but there are two wild fruits which can be used in the same ways. The Sierra (Pacific or Californian) Plum (Prunus subcordada) can be found in northern California and south Oregon. In the southern part of its range it tends to be smaller with a drier flavour and this is the type needed for sloe gin. The fleshier and sweeter fruits found in the north are better for preserving. The Porter's plum or Allegheny Sloe (Prunus alleghaniensis) can be found from Connecticut to the Pennsylvania mountains. It is slightly acid but sweeter than European sloes and can be used in the same ways.

Sloe and Apple Jelly

Sloes and apples make a light crimson jelly that goes well with scones and cream.

900g (2lbs) sloes
900g (2lbs) cooking apples
1.15 litres (2 pints) water
450g (1lb) light brown (demerara) sugar per 575ml (1 pint) juice

Put the sloes into a large saucepan or preserving pan. Chop the apples, without peeling or coring and put them with the sloes. Pour in the water. Set the pan on a low heat and bring the contents gently to the boil. Simmer, stirring frequently, until the fruits are very soft, about 45 minutes.

Pour the fruit pulp into a jelly bag and let the juice drip into a bowl. Return the juice to the cleaned pan and bring it to the boil. Stir in the sugar, let it dissolve and boil until setting point is reached.

Take the pan from the heat and skim the jelly. Pour it into warmed jars and cover it with circles of waxed greaseproof paper. Cover it completely when cold. Makes about 900g (2lbs).

Sloe Gin

Sloe gin is a warming, rich red liqueur, just right for drinking at Christmas and the New Year.

1 bottle gin
175g (6oz) sloes
125g (4oz) granulated sugar

Pour all the gin from the bottle. Prick the sloes all over with a fork and put them into the gin bottle. Cover them with the sugar and pour back as much gin as possible into the bottle. Put the cap on the bottle.

Turn the bottle upside down to start to dissolve the sugar and then leave it to stand. Do this every day for two months. Then let the bottle stand, undisturbed, for three weeks. After this, decant the gin into another bottle.

At this point, you can top up the sloes with more gin, filling the bottle again. Leave them undisturbed for two to three months and you will have a liqueur only slightly less rich than the first.

Sloe Vodka

This can be made in exactly the same way as sloe gin. It has a cleaner, fruitier flavour, but is just as rich.

Medicinal

A gentle purgative: Infuse 2.5ml (½ teaspoon) dried blackthorn flowers in 100ml (3½ fl oz) boiling water for 10 minutes. Strain. Drink the whole amount first thing in the morning on an empty stomach.

For diarrhoea and dysentery: Pick sloes before they are fully ripe. Boil 50g (2oz) in 1 litre (1¾ pints) water or red wine for 5 minutes. Remove them from the heat and let them stand for 10 minutes. Drink the whole amount throughout the day, one cupful at a time.

SLOE

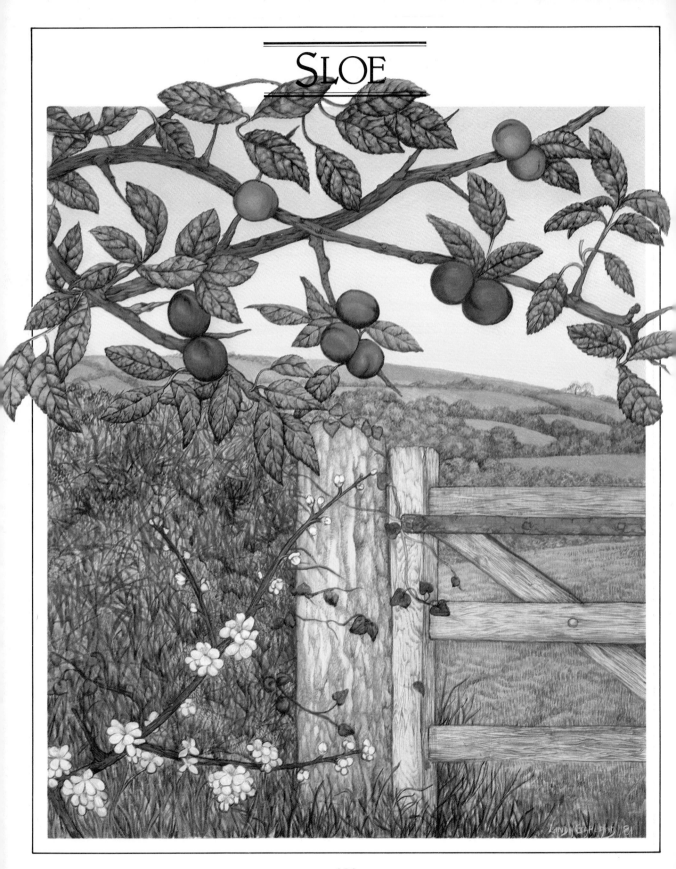

SWEET CHESTNUT

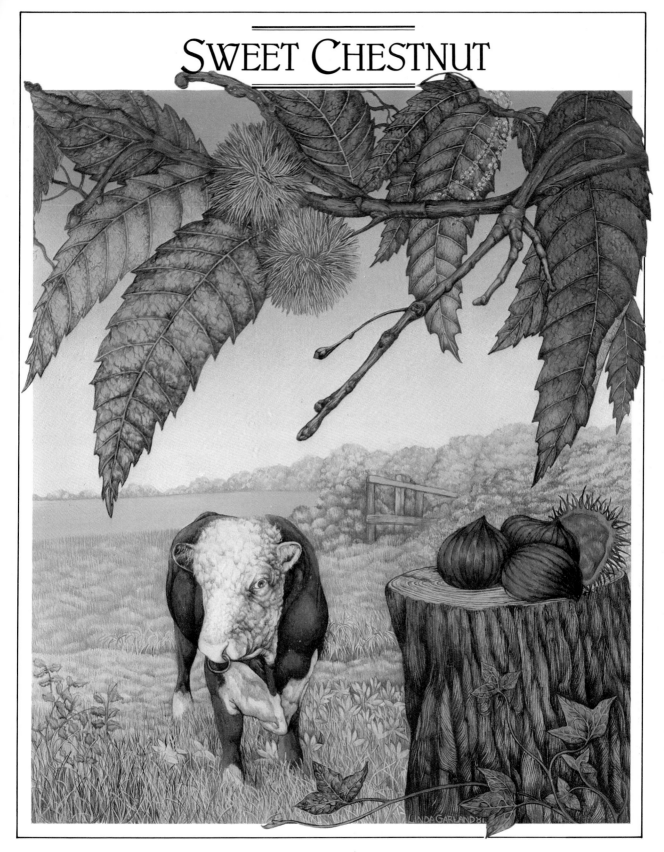

Availability

The sweet chestnut originated in the forests of southern Europe but it now grows throughout Europe, Scandinavia and Britain. It is less common in Scotland. It is mostly found in woodland but is often cultivated in parks and large gardens.

In the United States, the sweet or American chestnut (Castanea dentata) grows wild mainly in the eastern, mid-western and southern states. It is sadly becoming less common as it is being destroyed from the east by a fungal disease. The American chestnut is cultivated elsewhere in the United States.

Chestnuts start to drop from the trees in mid autumn (October in the northern hemisphere). At first, they will be completely covered by their prickly outer husk. To extract them, stamp on the husk and gently prize it apart. Later in the autumn, the husk will split as the nuts fall and you will be able to pick up the nuts from all round the tree.

Freshly gathered nuts, especially at the beginning of the season, taste sweet and milky when they are eaten raw. Make sure that you scrape away the furry inner skin as it is very bitter and drying. Keep the nuts in a cool place for a few days and they will be better for roasting and cooking.

Chestnut leaves for medicinal purposes should be picked in summer and dried.

To Roast Chestnuts

First of all you must slit the tops of the chestnuts or they will explode quite violently, whichever way you roast them. If you are preparing a good many, it is best to hold them on a chopping board. This prevents blunted knives and cut fingers. Slit the top sideways, without removing it completely.

To roast chestnuts in the oven, put them onto a baking sheet and into a preheated Reg 6/200C/400F oven for 15 minutes.

To roast them in the fire, wait until the fire dies down and the embers are still glowing. Put the chestnuts into the embers for about five minutes. Pick them out carefully, with tongs or a small shovel.

You can buy from some places that sell fire accessories (tongs, pokers, etc.) small chestnut roasters. They are like a small, cast iron frying pan with holes at regular intervals over the base and with a long handle. Slit the chestnuts, put them into the roaster and shake them over the hot fire for about 7 minutes.

A porcelain or terra cotta potato pot will also give excellent results. Put the slit chestnuts into the pot and leave them on a medium heat for 7–10 minutes, shaking them several times.

You can eat roast chestnuts while you are sitting round the fire on a winter's afternoon or evening. You can also serve them as a first course, accompanied with butter.

To store chestnuts

Layer them in dry sand, straw or tightly screwed up newspaper. They will keep for about three months.

Pork Knuckles with Chestnuts and Apples

225 g (8 oz) chestnuts
2 medium sized cooking apples
2 pork knuckles
2 medium onions, thinly sliced
575 ml (1 pint) dry cider
bouquet of parsley, sage, thyme and marjoram
sea salt and freshly ground black pepper

Heat the oven to Reg 4/180C/350F. Skin the chestnuts. Peel, core and chop the apples. Put the pork knuckles into a large, flameproof casserole. Surround them with the chestnuts, apples and onions. Pour in the cider, add the bouquet garni and season well. Set the casserole on a high heat and bring the cider to the boil. Cover the casserole and put it into the oven for 1½ hours.

Take out the pork knuckles. Remove the rinds and carve the meat. Put the meat into a serving dish and spoon the chestnuts and casserole juices over the top. The apples will have melted into the liquid. Serves 4.

To Skin Chestnuts

Slit the tops as for roasting. Put the chestnuts into a saucepan and cover them with cold water. Bring them to the boil and take them from the heat.

Skin them as soon as they have cooled enough to be handled, leaving them in the water until you get to them.

Lamb, Lemon and Chestnuts

Chestnuts cooked whole with meat become plump and soft and pick up all the flavours of the dish.

one shoulder lamb
225 g (8 oz) chestnuts
25 g (1 oz) butter
1 large onion, thinly sliced
275 ml (½ pint) stock
grated rind and juice 1 lemon
15 ml (1 tablespoon) chopped lemon thyme
15 ml (1 tablespoon) chopped marjoram

Bone the lamb and cut the meat into 2 cm (¾ inch) cubes. Skin the chestnuts. Melt the butter in a large, heavy frying pan or a sauté pan on a high heat. Put in the lamb, brown it well and remove it. Lower the heat. Put in the onion and soften it. Stir in the chestnuts and pour in the stock. Bring it gently to the boil. Add the lemon rind and juice and replace the lamb. Cover the pan and leave it on the lowest heat possible for 30 minutes. Serves 4.

Goose with Pork and Chestnut Stuffing

Apples, pork and chestnuts make a very light textured stuffing for goose.

one 4.5 kg (10 lb) goose
225 g (8 oz) chestnuts
450 g (1 lb) lean pork
75 g (3 oz) streaky bacon
15 g (½ oz) butter
1 large onion, finely chopped
1 large cooking apple, finely chopped
10 sage leaves, chopped
30 ml (2 tablespoons) chopped parsley
15 ml (1 tablespoon) wholewheat flour
275 ml (½ pint) dry cider
275 ml (½ pint) stock (made from the giblets)
45 ml (3 tablespoons) chopped parsley
6 sage leaves, chopped

Skin the chestnuts. Put them with the pork through the fine blade of a mincer. Put them into a mixing bowl. Dice the bacon. Melt the butter in a frying pan on a low heat. Put in the bacon and onion and cook them until the bacon is soft. Mix in the apple and continue cooking for 1 minute more. Mix the contents of the frying pan into the pork and chestnuts. Add the sage and parsley and mix well.

Heat the oven to Reg 6/200C/400F. Stuff and truss the goose. Put it on a rack in a roasting tin and cover it completely with foil. Put it into the oven for 2 hours. Remove the foil and cook for a further 30 minutes so the skin crisps and browns.

Take out the goose. Pour off any fat from the roasting tin and leave in any brown juices. Set the tin on top of the stove on a moderate heat. Stir in the flour and cook it for 1 minute. Pour in the cider and stock and bring them to the boil, stirring. Add the parsley and sage and simmer for 5 minutes.

Carve the goose at the table and serve the sauce separately. Serves 8.

Chestnut Shortbreads

These are softer than the usual shortbread biscuits. They are a real golden brown with a spiced nutty flavour.

175 g (6 oz) chestnuts
150 ml (¼ pint) milk
5 cm (2 inch) piece cinnamon stick
125 g (4 oz) butter
50 g (2 oz) honey
5 ml (1 teaspoon) ground cinnamon
175 g (6 oz) wholewheat flour

Heat the oven to Reg 4/180C/350F. Skin the chestnuts. Put them into a saucepan with the milk and cinnamon stick. Bring them gently to the boil and simmer them, covered, for 20 minutes so they are soft and all the milk has been absorbed.

Put the chestnuts into a mixing bowl and mash them with a potato masher. Cut the butter into small pieces and beat it into the chestnuts. Mix in the honey. Fold in the flour and bring the mixture together with your fingers to make a soft, workable dough.

Put the dough onto a floured work surface and roll it out to about 6 mm (¼ inch). Stamp it into rounds with a 6 cm (2½ inch) thick biscuit cutter. Lay the biscuits on a floured baking sheet and bake them for 15 minutes so they are golden brown but still soft. Using a palette knife, lift them carefully onto a wire rack so they cool and firm. Makes about 24.

Medicinal

For irritating coughs and whooping cough:
Infuse 25 g (1 oz) dried chestnut leaves in 575 ml (1
pint) boiling water for 10 minutes. Strain and
drink a small wineglassful three or four times a
day.

For asthma and other chest complaints: Boil
25 g (1 oz) fresh or 15 g (½ oz) dried chestnut
leaves in 850 ml (1½ pints) water for 10 minutes.
Strain and cool. Add 15 g (½ oz) honey and 15 g
(½ oz) glycerine. Drink 100 ml (3½ fl oz) on rising
and the same amount last thing at night.

Veterinary

Pigs are fond of chestnuts and chestnut-fed pork
is a meat of excellent quality.
To lure a pig to market, put down a trail of
chestnuts in front of him.
Dried chestnuts can be milled to make feed for
horses, cattle and pigs. If milled into smaller
pieces they can be fed to poultry and pigeons.
Fallen chestnut leaves can be used as litter for
calves, goats and chickens.

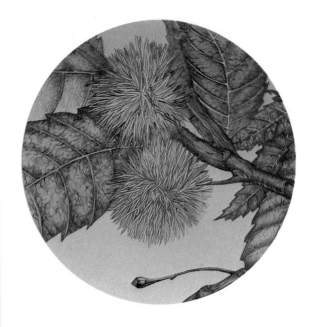

Bibliography

Bairacli Levi, Juliette de, *Herbal Handbook for Everyone*, Faber and Faber Ltd., 1966.

Bairacli, Levy, Juliette de, *Herbal Handbook for Farm and Stable*, Faber and Faber Ltd., 1973

Brackett, Babette; and Lash, Maryann, *The Wild Gourmet*, David R. Godine, Boston, 1975

Buchner, Greet, *Cooking with Flowers*, Thorson's Publishers Ltd., 1978

Ceres, *Herbs for Healthy Hair*, Thorson's Publishers Ltd., 1978

Crowhurst, Adrienne, *The Weed Cookbook*, Lancer Books, N.Y., 1972

Crowhurst, Adrienne, *The Flower Cookbook*, Lancer Books, N.Y., 1973

Edlin, H.L., *British Plants and Their Uses*, B.T. Batsford Ltd., 1951

Fitter, Richard; and Fitter, Alistair, *The Wild Flowers of Britain and Northern Europe*, Collins, 1974

Grieve, Mrs., *A Modern Herbal*, Penguin Books Ltd., 1976

Grigson, Geoffrey, *The Englishman's Flora*, Paladin, 1975

Harris, Ben Charles, *Eat the Weeds*, Barre Publishers, Mass., 1972

Hartley, Dorothy, *Food in England*, Macdonald, 1973

Howes, F.N., *Nuts, Their Production and Everyday Uses*, Faber and Faber, 1958

Jordan, Michael, *A Guide to Wild Plants*, Millington Books Ltd., 1976

Jordan, Michael, *A Guide to Mushrooms*, Millington Books Ltd., 1975

Kloss, Jethro, *Back to Eden*, Woodbridge Press Pub. Co., Calif., 1975

Lange, Morten; and Hora, F. Bayard, *Collins Guide to Mushrooms and Toadstools*, 1972

Leyel, Mrs. C.F., *The Magic of Herbs*, Jonathan Cape, 1926

Leyel, Mrs. C.F., *Compassionate Herbs*, Faber and Faber Ltd., 1946

Leyel, Mrs. C.F., *Hearts Ease*, Faber and Faber Ltd., 1949

Leyel, Mrs. C.F., *Herbal Delights*, Faber and Faber Ltd., 1937

Loewenfeld, Clare, *Britain's Wild Larder, Nuts*, Faber and Faber Ltd., 1967

Mabey, Richard, *Food for Free*, Collins 1972

MacNicol, Mary, *Flower Cookery*, Collier Books, N.Y., 1972

Medsger, Oliver Perry, *Edible Wild Plants*, Macmillan Publishing Co. Inc., N.Y., 1978

Miller, Orson K. Jnr., *Mushrooms of North America*, E.P. Dutton. N.Y., 1980

National Federation of Women's Institutes, *Lotions and Potions*

Palaiseul, Jean, *Grandmother's Secrets*, Penguin Books Ltd., 1973

Petulengro, Gypsy, *Romany Remedies and Recipes*, Methuen and Co. Ltd., 1935

Petulengro, Leon, *The Roots of Health*, Pan Books Ltd., 1968

Petulengro, Leon, *Herbs and Astrology*, Darton, Longman and Todd, 1977

Smith, William, *Wonders in Weeds*, Health Science Press, 1977

Thomson, William A.R., M.D., (ed) *Healing Plants, A Modern Herbal*, Macmillan London Ltd., 1980

Veissid, Jacques, *Folk Medicine*, Quartet Books, 1979

White, Florence, *Flowers as Food*, Jonathan Cape, 1934

Wiggington, Eliot, (ed) *Foxfire 2*, Anchor Press, N.Y., 1973

Wiggington, Eliot, (ed) *Foxfire 3*, Anchor Press, N.Y., 1975

Zeitlmayr, Linus, *Wild Mushrooms, an Illustrated Handbook*, Frederick Muller, 1968

Index